THE FRUGAL CARNIVORE DIET MADE EASY

Carnivore Diet Cookbook on a Low
Budget Including Eating Eggs, a
1 Week Meal Plan, and a 3 Day Meal Plan

DELICIOUS DELIGHTS PUBLISHING

THANK YOU FOR YOUR PURCHASE!

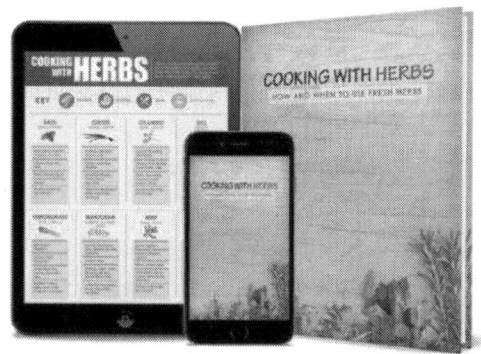

DO YOU LIKE DELICIOUS DELIGHTS PUBLISHING? SUBSCRIBE TO OUR NEWSLETTER AND DOWNLOAD YOUR FREE GIFT NOW!

DISCOVER SIMPLE HERB RECIPES TO ADD FLAVOR TO YOUR DRINKS AND COOKING! ENHANCE THE TASTE OF YOUR DRINKS AND DISHES!

https:// l.ead.me/ddp-free-gift

https:// l.ead.me/wb-free-gift

TABLE OF CONTENTS

Introduction to the Frugal Carnivore Diet 6

Butter Burgers 11

Pork Chops 14

Deli Roast Beef 17

Carnivore Waffles 20

Baked Ham & Egg 23

Carnivore Custard 25

Ham & Goat Cheese Frittata 27

Chicken Wings 29

Pickled Eggs 32

Bacon Egg Quiche 34

Egg Omelette 36

Poached Eggs 38

Scotch Eggs 40

Meatballs 42

Pork Belly 45

Ground Beef Casserole 47

Meat Muffins 49

Liver Pate 51

Lamb Chops 53

Bone Marrow Broth 56

Egg Smoked Salmon Crepes 58

Baked Salmon 60

Three Cheese Omelette 62

Butter Roasted Chicken 65

Cinnamon Butter Chicken Thigh 68

Organ Meat Burgers 70

Fish Cakes 73

Baked Fish 76

Grilled Tuna 79

Stir-Fried Beef Hearts 81

FOODS ALLOWED ON THE CARNIVORE DIET 83

INTRODUCTION TO THE FRUGAL CARNIVORE DIET

Do the thought of eating juicy, tender steaks and burger patties three times a day for an extended period without any veggies, grains, and fruits excite you? If you said yes, then the carnivore diet might be for you. The diet is similar to the food lifestyle on which the hunter-gatherer based their life. And it is for this reason; the carnivore diet is gaining prominence and becoming an upcoming food trend in recent years.

The carnivore diet is a zero-carb intense elimination diet that excludes all foods except animal products such as meat, eggs, and fish. Therefore, there aren't any vegetables, fruits, nuts, or seeds in this highly restrictive diet but just animals and their products. The founding belief concerning this diet is that carbohydrates are responsible for most chronic diseases like cancer etc. and therefore the diet revolves around food ingredients like beef, pork, lamb, chicken, fish, organ meats, eggs, bone marrow, bone broth, lard, etc. Furthermore, the diet emphasizes consuming fatter cuts of meat so that each meal can make you feel full while meeting your daily energy requirements. Staying hydrated through water and bone broth is encouraged since drinking coffee and tea should be kept to a minimum. It is considered an extension of the keto and paleo diets. It is mainly undertaken by those who have auto-immune conditions or any food insensitivities and want faster weight loss.

As the carnivore diet is similar to the keto diet, many dieters report identical benefits such as faster weight loss, improved bowel movements, enhanced skin health, better muscle growth and retention, and heightened focus. People consider it for weight loss most of the time, as the calories consumed will be less since only one food item, the meat is taken. And that, too, is a highly satiating one since it is protein-laden.

As protein and fat are the main components in meat, they leave less residue when absorbed in the small intestines. Thus, there is a possibility of getting constipated, especially during the first few weeks as they are fewer leftovers that can irritate the gut and which in turn help to rebuild and recover the gut. For this reason, this type of low-residue diet can be helpful for those who have symptoms of inflammatory bowel disease and irritable bowel syndrome that are triggered by plant fibers and other compounds.

What's more, the diet proponents claim a lower level of inflammatory conditions in the body while boosting energy levels and overall health. However, they aren't any long-term scientific studies on this diet yet.

The diet is much simple to follow than keto and other diets as you don't have to calculate calories, track your macros, or be concerned about what meals are okay and whether you're over your carb limit. You eat meat and go on with your day. For this reason, following this diet is an absolute breeze.

On the other hand, the downside of following this diet is that there is a possibility of nutritional deficiencies. For example, Vitamin C and E intake will drop significantly in the diet as plant food rich in various nutrients is forbidden. But it is also to be noted that with reduced glucose, the need for it also decreases. Next, the chances of gut microbiome damage are high. Though improved digestive health is touted as a benefit of this diet, nutritionists fear that those benefits are short-term and are mainly an outcome of eliminating inflammatory foods. As a result, both good and harmful ones are removed from the system. The third side effect is the higher percentage of excess sodium and saturated fats in these foods. Eating only meat products and dairy can cause a surge in sodium intake, leading to headaches, swelling, and kidney disease.

Because the diet is concerned with the higher consumption of red meat, there would be a higher possibility of excess saturated fat, which has been linked to an increased risk of stroke and gastric cancer. Lastly, solid cravings for other food items and boredom of eating the same food day after day can cause undue stress. The more restrictive a diet is, the more will be your cravings. Being not able to enjoy fruits and vegetables is too hard. You would have to test your willpower against the restrictive items repeatedly. Eating meat alone can be tedious.

TIPS FOR FOLLOWING THE CARNIVORE DIET

Starting a new diet can be a bit overwhelming and can backfire when not done correctly. Therefore, any tips from those who have done the diet successfully can help you stay strong in this diet are:

- Consume grass-fed meats whenever possible. Grass-fed and pasture-raised meat are much more beneficial since the meat will absorb more nutrients from the grass, which is healthier for you.

- Try the diet for a month or two, and then see how your body is getting accustomed to the diet. Based on that, you can progress forward. Based on your health conditions and your goals, you can determine which level of carnivore diet you want to go for.

- Enjoy the food you are eating rather than being anxious about whether you are doing it right or wrong. Stress can cause problems for food digestion, and it is vital for healthy eating. Therefore avoid stress at all costs. For example, concerning spices, you can be a bit relaxed initially, and once you are into the diet, you can start eliminating the ones that are prohibited in the diet.

- Make sure to comprise offal and other organ meats in your diet as they constitute the most nutrient-dense foods. When we incorporate these ingredients into your diet, it will give you a change from the usual carnivore diet and make sure your body is getting its critical nutrients. But then it is not essential to include them at the beginning, especially if you haven't had them before.

- Make sure to include natural, unprocessed salt in your diet so as to manage your hydration level. Once carbohydrates are eliminated from your diet, there is a high possibility of losing stored water. With the salt added, the mineral balance gets corrected, and you will feel all energized.

- Try to understand how your body is reacting to the diet. Notice your body and pay close attention to how you feel. If it works for you, great, but if you are miserable and feel weak and aren't getting any of the benefits, you need to stop immediately.

- Be clear about why you want to start on this diet and the reason behind the decision to begin the carnivore diet. Once clarified about the 'why,' you will be able to progress successfully in the diet.

- You need to expect a bumpy start. For example, people usually suffer from an odd week of bowel movements before getting them back to normal. So with such a drastic variation to your diet, you need to expect things to get a bit weird.

- Consider it as a trial. As we don't have much scientific evidence on the long-term effects of carnivore diets, there are risks. The carnivore may be healthy for the first months but harmful for more extended periods. Or it could also be beneficial in perpetuity.

- Test your blood work frequently. When periodical check-ups are done on your blood, you will notice any alarming spikes that may arise from swapping your diet so dramatically.

- Taking multivitamins can be beneficial to overcome any nutritional deficiency if any.

- If possible, plan ahead and make a meal plan for the week, as meal prep can aid you to stay ahead of time and stick to it. Writing down your meal plan and cooking snacks and meals ahead of time will significantly increase your chances of successfully sticking with the carnivore diet.

- Now that you have all the essential information about the frugal carnivore diet, you can carefully consider and check whether this diet is suitable for you. For example, under no conditions should people who suffer from kidneys be allowed. But then, it would always be helpful to consult your family physician and understand whether the diet is ideal for you.

BUTTER BURGERS

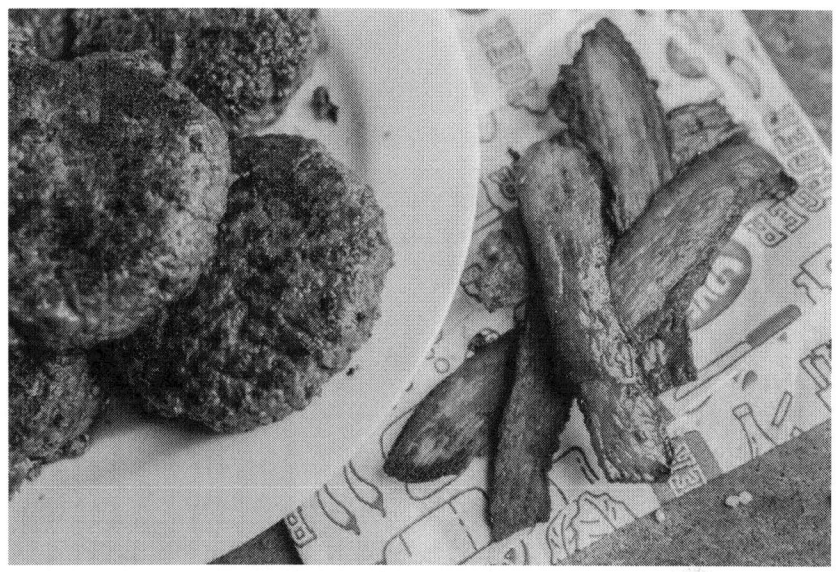

A wholesome, savory dish that comes together quickly for weekday dinner is always a keeper! On top of it, the combo of beef, gooey cheese, and butter makes it juicy and cheesy while exploding it with tons of buttery flavor and taste.

Preparation Time: 10 Minutes

Cooking Time: 10 Minutes

Serving Size: 12

Ingredients:

- 1 lb. Beef, ground & 85% lean
- Grounded Black Pepper, to taste
- Garlic Powder, as needed & optional
- 3 tbsp. Butter

- Sea Salt, to taste

- 2 oz. Cheese

Method of Preparation:

1. Preheat the oven to 375 ° F or 190 ° C.

2. After that, season the ground beef with salt and pepper in a medium-sized bowl. If using garlic powder, spoon it in.

3. Then, place about one tablespoon of beef into the bottom of a greased muffin pan. Tip: The meat should fully cover the bottom.

4. Now, spoon in a pat of butter on top of the beef pieces and add beef to the top. Press gently to flatten.

5. Now, keep a small piece of cheese to the beef and add a final layer of beef.

6. Bake for 10 minutes, and once the time is up, open the door slightly for 5 to 10 minutes. Tip: This will allow the excess oil to cool down.

7. Remove from the pan from the oven and serve them warm.

Tip: If you prefer, you can add onion powder to it for more flavor.

Serving Suggestion: The butter beef burgers are delicious on their own. Or they can be served on top of simple green salad based on whether you are following the strict carnivore diet or not.

Storage Suggestion: Store them in an air-tight container for up to 5 days in the refrigerator

Nutritional Information per Serving:

- **Calories**: 125Kcal
- **Fat**: 10g
- **Carbohydrates**: 0g
- **Proteins**: 8g

PORK CHOPS

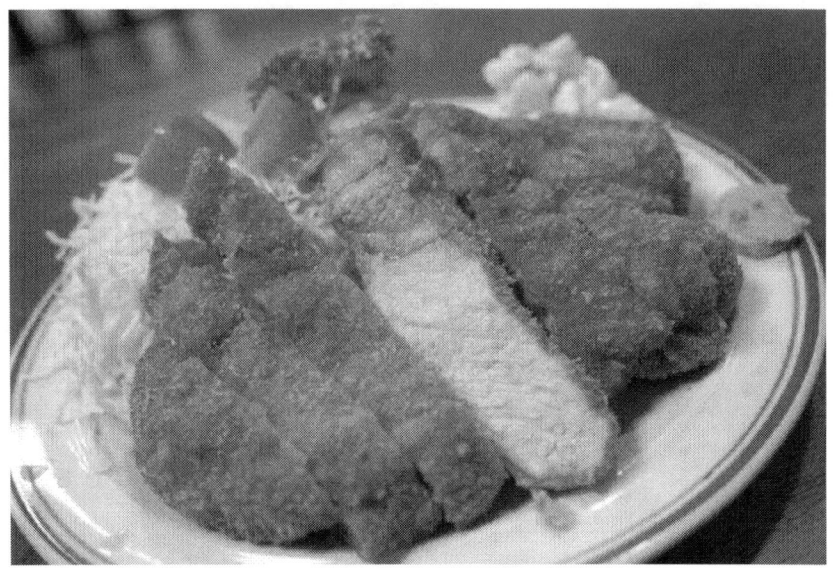

These tender pork chops with a crispy, cheesy outer coating and juicy insides are a tasty way to enjoy the pork meat. Furthermore, since it is made in the air fryer, it takes less than 40 minutes to bring it to the table.

Preparation Time: 10 Minutes

Cooking Time: 30 Minutes

Serving Size: 4

Ingredients:

- 5 oz. Pork Chops, boneless

- 1 tbsp. Heavy Whipping Cream

- 1 tsp. Pink Himalayan Salt

- 2 Eggs, large

- 1 cup Pork Rinds, grounded

- ¼ tsp. Black Pepper

- ¾ cup Parmesan Cheese, grated

- ½ tsp. Garlic Powder, optional

- 1 tsp. Paprika, optional

- ½ tsp. Onion Powder, optional

Method of Preparation:

1. First, with paper towels, pat the pork chops until dry.

2. Marinate the pork chops on both sides with salt and pepper.

3. After that, mix parmesan, salt, pork rinds, and black pepper in a large-sized shallow bowl. Tip: Add the seasoning if using at this stage.

4. Then, beat egg and cream in another bowl until combined.

5. Now, dredge the chops in the egg-cream mixture first and then coat it in the crumb mixture. Keep it aside.

6. Preheat the air fryer at 400°F or 200 ° C for 3 minutes.

7. Once hot, arrange the coated pork chops in the greased air-fryer basket.

8. Cook for 12 to 14 minutes while flipping it halfway through the baking time. Tip: The internal temperature should reach at least 145 ° F for rare to 155 ° F for well done.

9. Finally, take the chops from the air fryer and keep them

aside to rest for few minutes.

10. Serve them warm.

Tip: If you prefer, you can add about one to two teaspoons of Italian seasoning to it for more flavor.

Serving Suggestion: The pork chops are delicious on their own. Or they can be served along with steamed broccoli or your choice of veggie, depending on whether you are following the carnivore diet completely or not.

Storage Suggestion: Store pork chops in an air-tight container for 3 to 4 days in the refrigerator.

Nutritional Information per Serving:

- **Calories**: 399Kcal

- **Fat**: 10g

- **Carbohydrates**: 2g

- **Proteins**: 46g

DELI ROAST BEEF

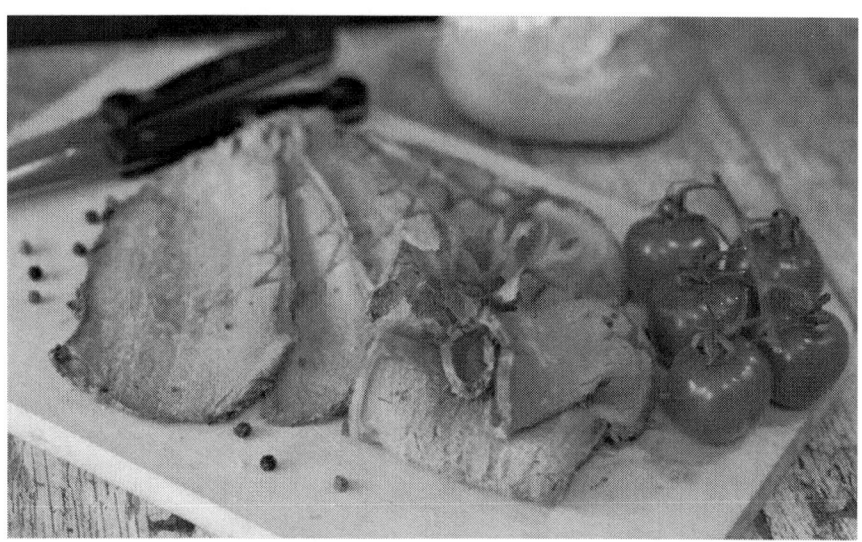

This super-tender roast beef is so much better than the store-bought ones with zero net carbs and no preservatives. What's more, it is so easy to simple and easy to make while being cooked to tender perfection.

Preparation Time: 10 Minutes

Cooking Time: 1 Hour 10 Minutes

Serving Size: 6

Ingredients:

- 3 lb. Bottom Round Beef Roast

- 2 tsp. Salt

- 2 tsp. Rosemary, fresh & finely chopped

- 1 tsp. Black Pepper, freshly grounded

- 2 tbsp. Olive Oil

- 1 tsp. Garlic Powder, optional

Method of Preparation:

1. Start by mixing garlic powder, if using salt, pepper, rosemary, and olive oil in a small-sized bowl.

2. Take out the meat from the refrigerator and coat it with marinade evenly over the meat surface. Set it out for 1 hour.

3. Roast for 60 to 90 minutes at 325 ° F or 162 ° C. Tip: The baking time depends on the roast size and the oven temperature. An instant-read thermometer inserted at the center after 50 minutes should be around 125 to 130 °F for medium-rare or 135 to 140° F for medium.

4. Allow the meat to cool completely before cutting into thin slices. Tip: If time permits, allow it to cool for a minimum of 30 minutes or for a maximum period of 2 to 3 hours.

5. Serve it thinly across the grain and enjoy.

Tip: If you like to eat it cold, trim off any excess fat.

Serving Suggestion: The deli roast beef is delicious on its own. Or the beef can be smeared with cream cheese and rolled up.

Storage Suggestion: Cover them in foil or butcher paper and store them in an air-tight container in the refrigerator for four days.

Nutritional Information per Serving:

- **Calories**: 452Kcal

- **Fat**: 30g

- **Carbohydrates**: 0g
- **Proteins**: 43g

CARNIVORE WAFFLES

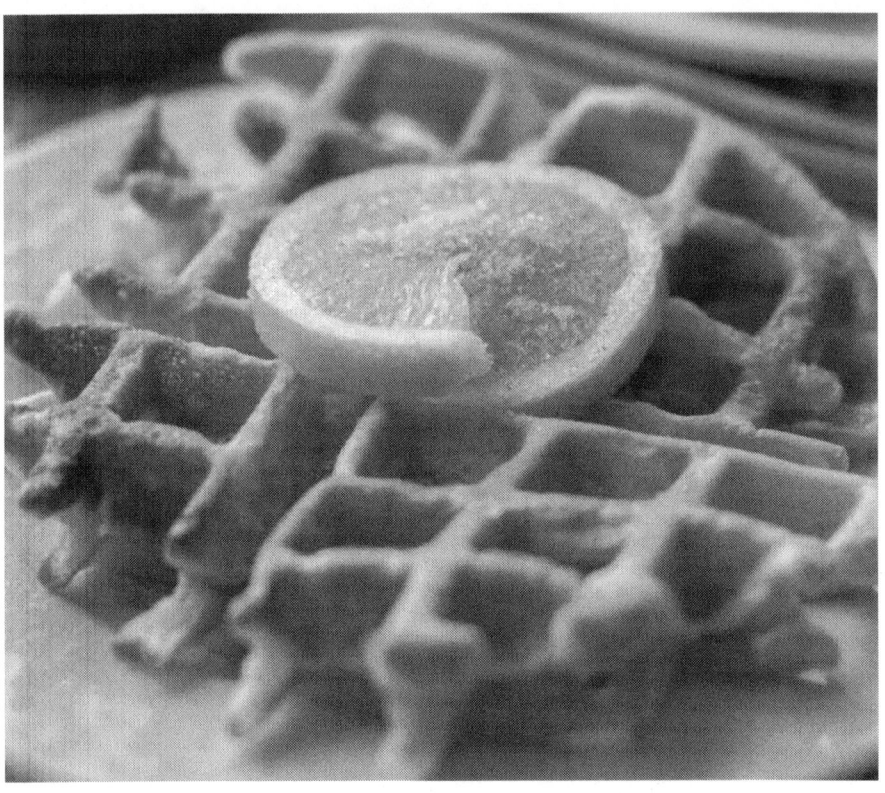

When you feel you need a change from the oh-so usual steaks and burgers, this paffle or carnivore waffle can be an excellent option to try out, especially when you miss the carb-rich waffles. On top, the carnivore waffles are a cinch to whip up, even on busy weeknights.

Preparation Time: 10 Minutes

Cooking Time: 10 Minutes

Serving Size: 2

Ingredients:

- 1 Egg
- Dash of Salt
- ½ cup Mozzarella Cheese
- ½ cup Pork Rinds, crushed

Method of Preparation:

1. First, preheat the waffle maker to medium-high heat.
2. Next, place pork rinds, cheese, salt, and egg in a large-sized mixing bowl and combine them with a whisker or place them in a blender and blend. Tip: The mixture should be smooth.
3. Once mixed well, pour the batter to the center of the waffle iron.
4. Close the waffle maker and allow it to cook for 4 to 5 minutes or until they are golden brown and cooked.
5. Serve and enjoy.

Tip: Instead of pork rinds, you can use ground beef.

Serving Suggestion: The carnivore waffle is delicious on its own. Or it can be paired with a pat of butter or runny egg on top along with French onion dip.

Storage Suggestion: Place all the waffles in a sheet pan while leaving ample space in between and freeze them for 30 minutes. Then, store them with parchment paper between each of them in a freezer-friendly bag. Reheat in the toaster for 4 minutes.

Nutritional Information per Serving:

- **Calories**: 270Kcal

- **Fat**: 19g

- **Carbohydrates**: 1.3g

- **Proteins**: 24.7g

BAKED HAM & EGG

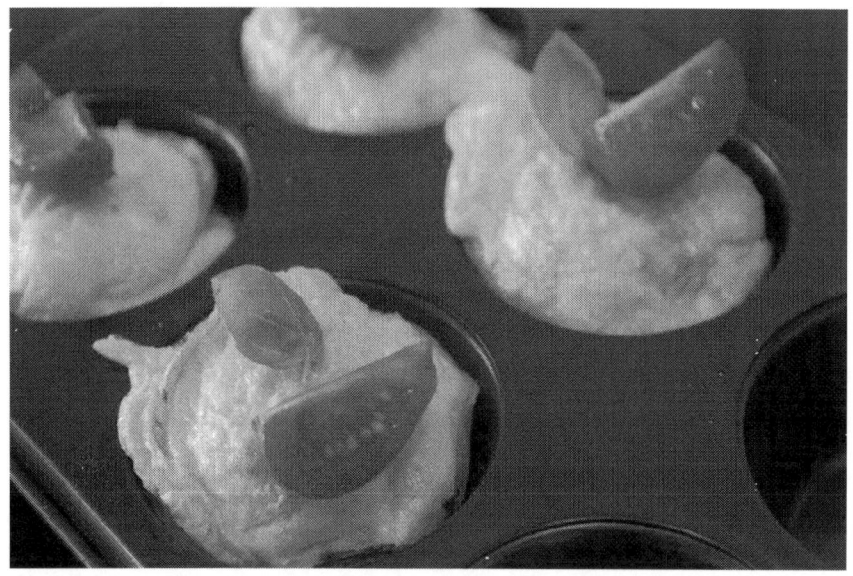

With the ham crispy around the edges and the eggs baking up fluffy, these protein-packed baked egg cups are the best of all standby dishes. They are ready in minutes and can be made from ingredients that you already have. To boot, every bite of these cups is sure to satisfy you with its texture and taste.

Preparation Time: 15 Minutes

Cooking Time: 15 Minutes

Serving Size: 6

Ingredients:

- 12 Ham Slices

- Sea Salt, as needed

- 6 Eggs, large

- ½ cup Milk, full-fat

- 1 tbsp. Thyme, optional

- Black Pepper, as needed

Method of Preparation:

1. Preheat the oven to 370 ° F or 185 ° C.

2. Then, place the ham slices in each of the muffin pan cups to cover it completely on all sides.

3. After that, mix egg, milk, black pepper, salt, and thyme if using in a large mixing bowl until combined well.

4. Now, pour the egg mixture into the molds evenly.

5. Finally, bake them for 14 to 15 minutes or until the eggs are cooked and the ham is crispy. Keep it aside for 5 minutes to cool slightly.

6. Serve them warm and enjoy.

Tip: If you prefer the egg to be runny, you need to bake them on for 12 minutes or so.

Serving Suggestion: The baked ham egg is delicious on its own.

Storage Suggestion: Store the leftovers in an air-tight container for 2 to 3 days. Reheat in the microwave for 30 to 40 seconds.

Nutritional Information per Serving:

- **Calories**: 340Kcal

- **Fat**: 30g

- **Carbohydrates**: 3g

- **Proteins**: 13g

CARNIVORE CUSTARD

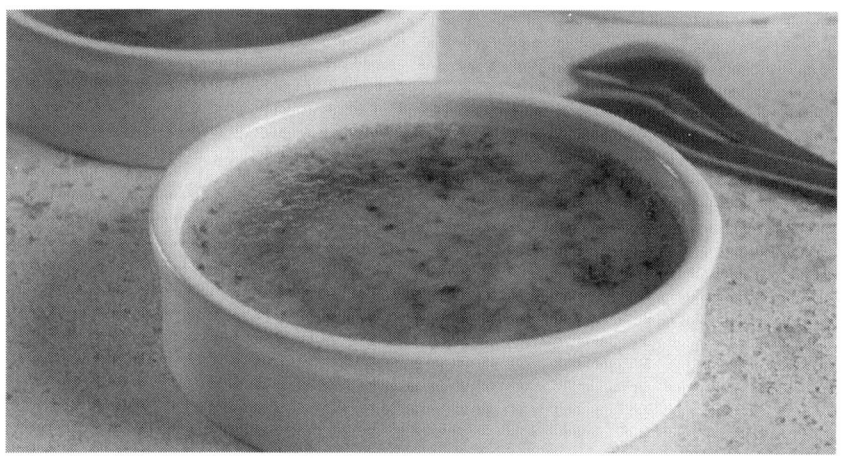

The best carnivore dessert comes to you through this easy and simple recipe. Sweet, creamy, and velvety thick, this positively divine custard is a treat you should frequently make as it will be a hit among kids and adults.

Preparation Time: 10 Minutes

Cooking Time: 30 Minutes

Serving Size: 4

Ingredients:

- 2 cups Heavy Cream

- 3 Eggs, whole

- 1 tbsp. Vanilla Extract, optional

Method of Preparation:

1. To begin with, preheat the oven to 350 ° F or 175 ° C.

2. After that, combine egg, heavy cream, and vanilla extract

if using in a large mixing bowl with a whisker.

3. Once mixed well, transfer the mixture to ramekins evenly and arrange them on a baking sheet.

4. Then, pour 3 cups of water into a medium-sized saucepan over medium heat and bring the water to a boil.

5. Add the water to the baking dish and place them in the lower rack of the oven.

6. Now, keep the ramekins in the oven and bake for half an hour, or until the custard top portion is set and golden brown. Tip: The bottom part will be slightly wiggly.

7. Remove the custard from the oven and set them aside for 1o to 15 minutes to cool. Tip: It will firm up with more time.

8. Serve them warm and enjoy.

Tip: You can also serve them cold.

Serving Suggestion: The carnivore egg custard is delicious on its own, or you can serve it on top of berries.

Storage Suggestion: Store the custard in an air-tight container for a week in the refrigerator. Or you store the ramekins in an air-tight container.

Nutritional Information per Serving:

- **Calories**: 421Kcal

- **Fat**: 44g

- **Carbohydrates**: 3g

- **Proteins**: 4g

HAM & GOAT CHEESE FRITTATA

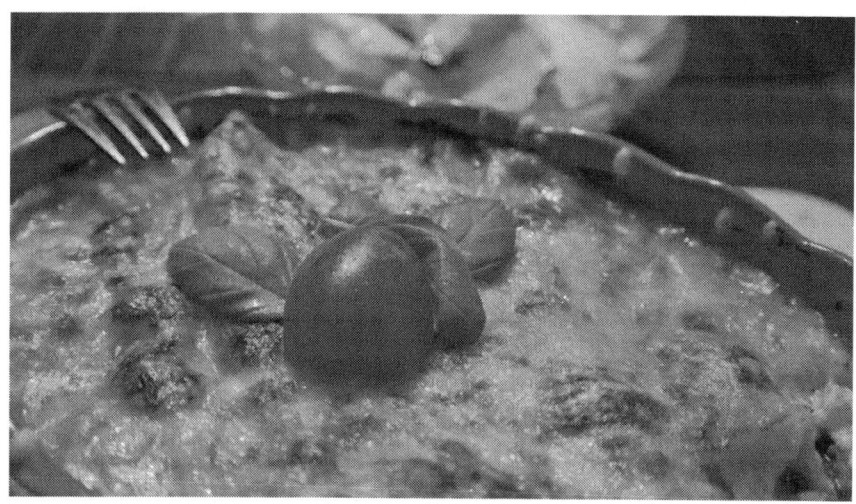

Don't you just love it when few simple ingredients come together to create an extraordinary tasty fare? If yes, then this dish creamy goat cheese paired with cheddar cheese and ham is a total delight to have.

Preparation Time: 10 Minutes

Cooking Time: 20 Minutes

Serving Size: 6

Ingredients:

- ½ cup Cheddar Cheese, grated

- ¼ cup Heavy Cream

- ½ tsp. Garlic Powder, optional

- 8 Eggs, large

- 6 oz. Ham, chopped

- 4 oz. Goat Cheese

Method of Preparation:

1. First, preheat the oven to 400 ° F or 200 ° C.

2. After that, place the eggs in a large-sized mixing bowl and beat the egg well with a whisker.

3. To this, spoon in the heavy cream and chopped ham.

4. Once mixed, stir in the cheddar cheese and garlic powder if using.

5. Now, transfer the mixture to a wide glass container and spread it across evenly.

6. Finally, bake for 15 minutes or until cooked.

7. Serve them warm and

Tip: If preferred, you can add crumbled bacon to it,

Serving Suggestion: The goat cheese frittata is delicious on its own.

Storage Suggestion: Store the frittata in an air-tight container for up to two to three days. Make sure to store them within 2 to 3 hours after cooking. You can pair it with a simple green salad or with bread.

Nutritional Information per Serving:

- **Calories**: 290Kcal

- **Fat**: 22g

- **Carbohydrates**: 0.5g

- **Proteins**: 20g

CHICKEN WINGS

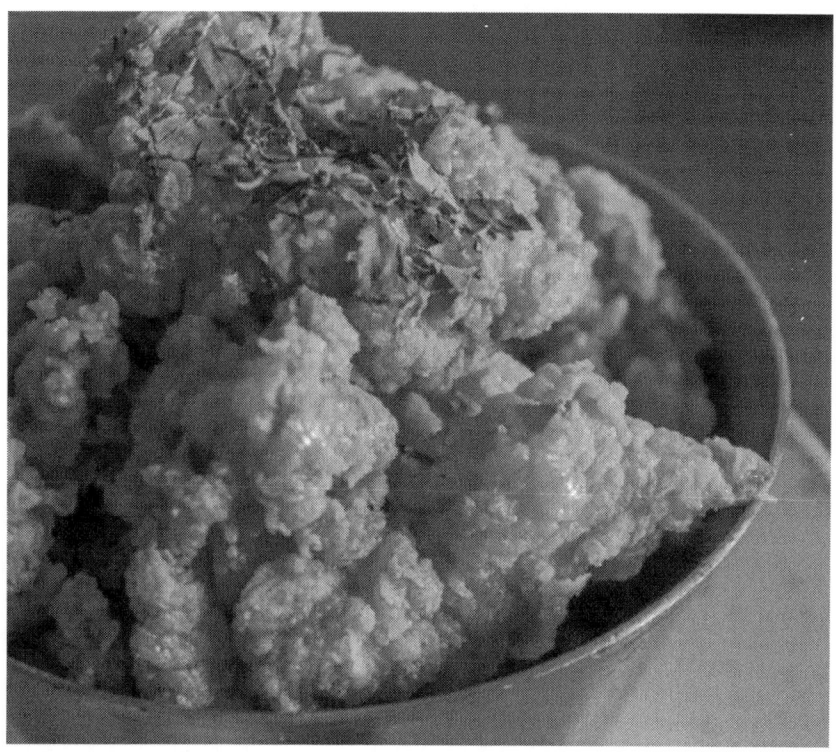

There is nothing better than these carnivore-diet-styled chicken wings. Crispy and finger-licking good; these chicken wings with the perfect crunch are so easy to make. What's more, the parmesan cheese adds a unique bite to the wings as it melts and crisps up in the oven, making them positively scrumptious.

Preparation Time: 10 Minutes

Cooking Time: 1 Hour

Serving Size: 8

Ingredients:

- 4 lb. Chicken Wings

- ¼ cup Butter, preferably grass-fed & softened

- ½ cup Parmesan, grated

- 1 tsp. Sea Salt

- ½ tsp. Black Pepper

Method of Preparation:

1. For making these tasty chicken wings, you need to first preheat the oven to 350 ° F or 175 ° C.

2. Next, place the butter in a large-sized mixing bowl and soften it well.

3. In another bowl, combine black pepper, cheese, and salt.

4. Now, coat the chicken pieces first in the butter and then in the cheese mix.

5. Then, arrange the chicken pieces in a parchment-paper-lined baking sheet while leaving ample space in between.

6. Finally, bake for 57 to 60 minutes or until they are golden browned and crispy.

7. Serve them warm and enjoy.

Tip: If preferred and allowed in your carnivore diet, you can add parsley to the recipe for more flavor.

Serving Suggestion: The baked chicken wings are delicious on their own. Or they can be paired with Blue cheese dip.

Storage Suggestion: Store the chicken wings in an air-tight container for up to four days. Make sure to store them within 2 to 3 hours after cooking.

Nutritional Information per Serving:

- **Calories**: 348Kcal
- **Fat**: 27g
- **Carbohydrates**: 1g
- **Proteins**: 25g

PICKLED EGGS

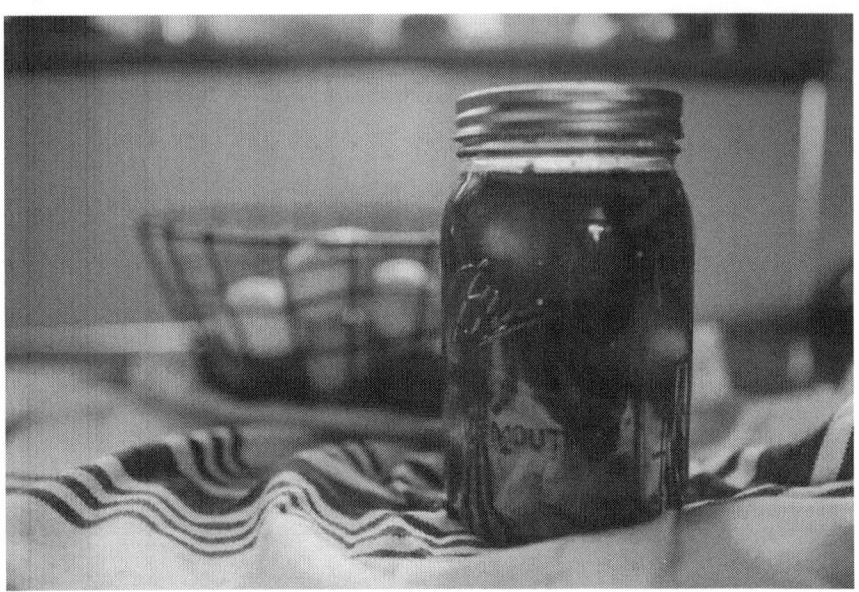

Great to snack on, these tangy and salty pickled eggs are excellent as appetizers. Furthermore, they don't require any canning and just use a simple brine concoction to make these prized eggs.

Preparation Time: 10 Minutes

Cure Time: 2 Days

Serving Size: 8

Ingredients:

- 8 Hard-boiled Eggs, large

- 2 tbsp. Pickling Spice

- 1 cup Water

- 1 tsp. Salt

- ½ cup Apple Cider Vinegar, raw

Method of Preparation:

1. Place the eggs, pickling spice, vinegar, salt, and water in a large pot and heat it over medium heat.

2. Bring to a gentle boil for 4 minutes. Set it aside for few minutes to cool.

3. Now, place the eggs in a large wide glass bottle or jar and pour the liquid over it.

4. Close the jar and keep it in the refrigerator for a minimum of two days or a maximum of seven days.

5. Serve and enjoy.

Tip: For a spicy version of a pickled egg, add one sliced jalapeno pepper to the jar.

Serving Suggestion: The pickled eggs is delicious on their own. Or they can be served along with deli meats as a light meal.

Storage Suggestion: Store the pickled eggs in an air-tight container with a tight lid in the refrigerator for up to a month.

Nutritional Information per Serving:

- **Calories**: 85Kcal
- **Fat**: 5g
- **Carbohydrates**: 2g
- **Proteins**: 6g

BACON EGG QUICHE

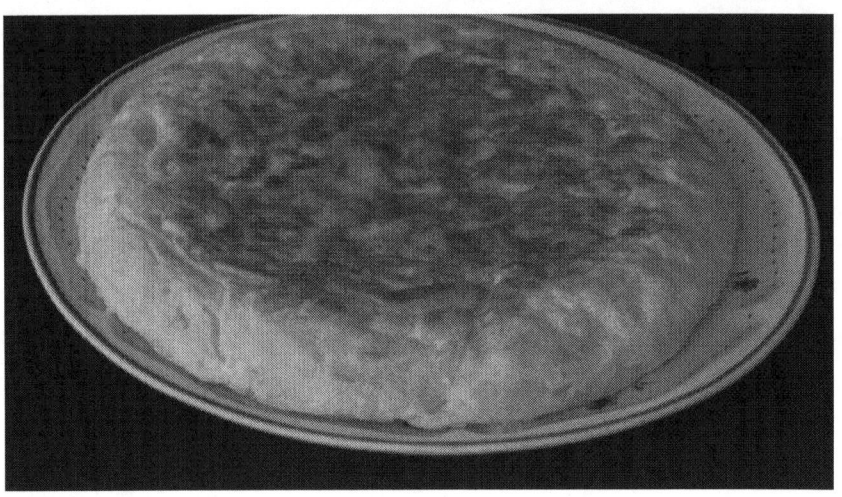

If you like to hear, people raving about how good your food is, then make these delicious quiches every now and then. Similar to the flavors of the breakfast sandwich, the combo of crispy bacon and salty cheese in the quiche brings on a winning combination that you would love. So make them soon without delay.

Preparation Time: 15 Minutes

Cooking Time: 45 Minutes

Serving Size: 12

Ingredients:

- 1 cup Heavy Whipping Cream
- 3 cups Cheddar Cheese, grated
- 12 Eggs
- 1 lb. Bacon, cooked & roughly chopped

Method of Preparation:

1.   Start by preheating the oven to 350 ° F or 175 ° C.

2.   Next, whisk the eggs and heavy cream in a large mixing bowl until combined well.

3.   Then, add the bacon and cheese to it and give everything a good stir.

4.   Once mixed well, transfer the mixture to a greased parchment-paper-lined baking sheet. Spread evenly.

5.   Finally, bake them for 30 to 35 minutes or until set and cooked. Tip: You can check for doneness with a toothpick. Insert in the center portion and see if it comes clean. If not, cook for some more time.

6.   Serve and enjoy.

Tip: If preferred and allowed, you can add thyme leaves to it for more flavor.

Serving Suggestion: The quiche is delicious on its own. Or you can serve it along with sour cream.

Storage Suggestion: Store the quiche in an air-tight container with a tight lid in the refrigerator for up to two to four days.

Nutritional Information per Serving:

- **Calories**: 310Kcal

- **Fat**: 26g

- **Carbohydrates**: 2g

- **Proteins**: 17g

EGG OMELETTE

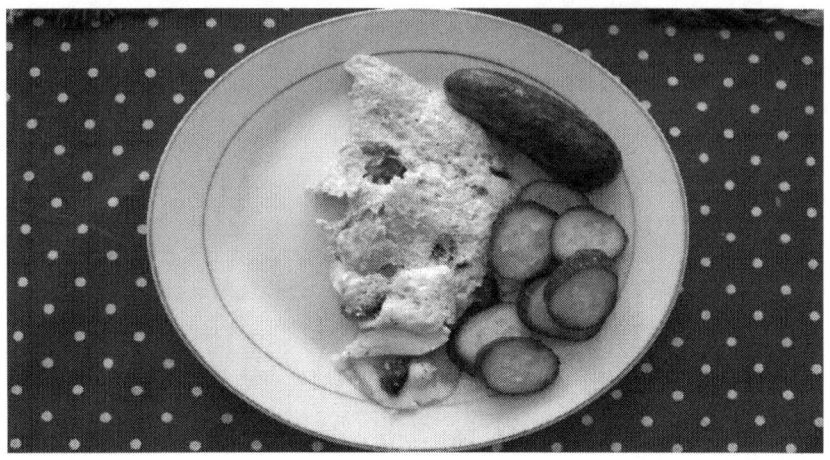

Absolutely flavorful, this protein-packed omelet has few simple ingredients 'married' to one another to create a flavor explosion. On top of it, it is a family-friendly recipe that makes a welcome breakfast meal or dinner.

Preparation Time: 5 Minutes

Cooking Time: 15 Minutes

Serving Size: 1 to 2

Ingredients:

- 4 Eggs, large
- ½ tsp. Sea Salt
- 1 Bacon
- 2 oz. Ground Beef
- 1 Salami
- 1 ½ tbsp. Mozzarella Cheese

Method of Preparation:

1. To begin with, place the bacon and ground beef in a heated pan over medium-high heat.

2. Continue cooking until browned and then transfer them to a plate.

3. Whisk eggs and salt in a large mixing bowl.

4. Next, pour the egg mixture into the pan and cook evenly on all sides. Tilt the pan so that all the portions are equally cooked.

5. Now, add the cooked and crumbled bacon, minced beef, ham, and mozzarella cheese on top of it and fold.

6. Serve them warm and enjoy.

Tip: You can add cold butter while whisking the egg to enhance the flavor and texture of the omelet.

Serving Suggestion: The omelet is delicious on its own. Or you can serve it along with sour cream.

Storage Suggestion: Store the omelet in an air-tight container with a tight lid in the refrigerator for up to two days.

Nutritional Information per Serving:

- **Calories**: 458Kcal

- **Fat**: 30g

- **Carbohydrates**: 2g

- **Proteins**: 45g

POACHED EGGS

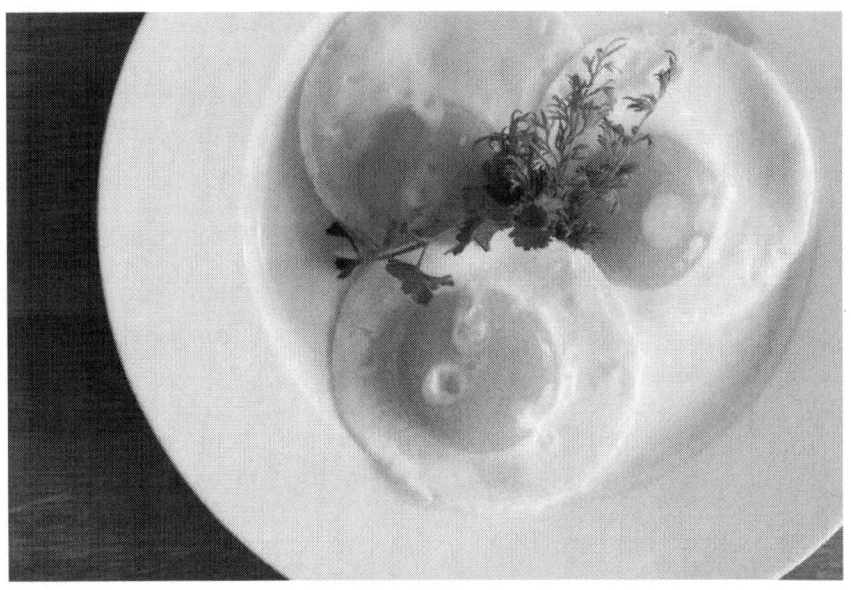

Though pouched egg may seem like a usual fare, this buttered poached egg is an indulgent dish as they are extra-rich in flavor and taste. What's more, the buttery taste gets soaked by the eggs and lends it a robust bite which is so good.

Preparation Time: 5 Minutes

Cooking Time: 10 Minutes

Serving Size: 1

Ingredients:

- 2 Eggs, large

- 4 tbsp. Butter

- ½ tsp. Black Pepper

- ½ tsp. Salt

Method of Preparation:

1. To begin with, heat a large skillet over medium-high heat.

2. Once it becomes hot, spoon in the butter and melt it.

3. Now, crack the eggs into it and cook for 3 to 5 minutes or until cooked. Tip: Do this slowly so that the egg does not spill out. The egg yolk should have a light white top.

4. Season it with salt and pepper.

5. Serve it warm and enjoy.

Tip: If you prefer, you can cook them for more than 6 minutes for a more cooked yolk.

Serving Suggestion: The poached egg is delicious on its own. Or top it with mozzarella cheese.

Storage Suggestion: Store the poached egg in an air-tight container with a tight lid in the refrigerator for up to a day.

Nutritional Information per Serving:

- **Calories**: 138Kcal

- **Fat**: 10g

- **Carbohydrates**: 1g

- **Proteins**: 11g

SCOTCH EGGS

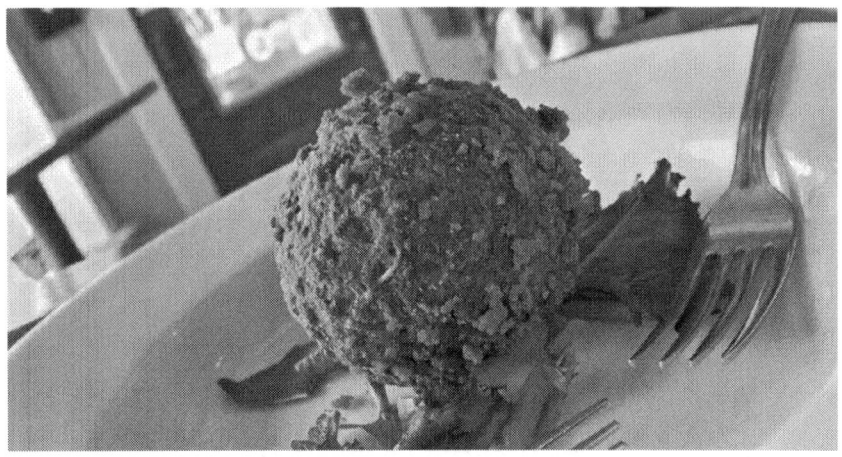

Are you stuck in a rut about what to make for breakfast while you are on the carnivore diet? Then these scotch eggs are an ideal fare to consider. Done well and done properly, it is easy to see why these cooked eggs coated in grounded beef are such a classic. The coalescence of the meaty grounded beef with the eggs results in a hearty meal that is bright and bursting with flavor.

Preparation Time: 15 Minutes

Cooking Time: 20 Minutes

Serving Size: Makes 12 Scotch Eggs

Ingredients:

- 2 lb. Beef, grounded

- 12 Hard-boiled Eggs

- 2 tsp. Salt

Method of Preparation:

1. First, preheat the oven to 350 ° F or 175 ° C.

2. After that, mix the ground beef and salt in a large mixing bowl until combined well.

3. Then, make 12 balls out of the beef mixture with your hands.

4. Now, arrange six balls on a greased parchment-paper-lined baking sheet and flatten them.

5. Next, place the eggs in the center portion and cover them entirely with the ground beef mixture. Tip: There shouldn't be any holes.

6. Finally, bake them for 13 to 15 minutes or until cooked.

7. Serve it warm and enjoy.

Tip: If desired, you can add a teaspoon of garlic powder for more flavor.

Serving Suggestion: The scotch eggs are delicious on their own. Or you can serve it along with sour cream.

Storage Suggestion: Store the scotch eggs in an air-tight container with a tight lid in the refrigerator for up to two days.

Nutritional Information per Serving:

- **Calories**: 270Kcal

- **Fat**: 20g

- **Carbohydrates**: 1g

- **Proteins**: 19g

MEATBALLS

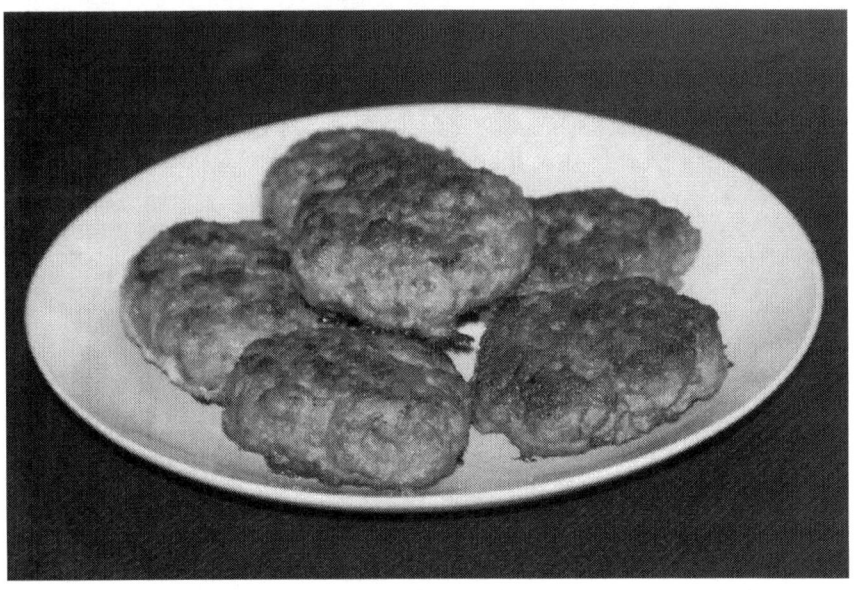

Amazingly tender all the way and deliciously flavorful, these baked meatballs made with ground pork, egg, parmesan cheese, and salt are sure to impress your family with their taste and texture. They are indeed comforting food at its best while being healthy.

Preparation Time: 5 Minutes

Cooking Time: 25 Minutes

Serving Size: 4

Ingredients:

- 2 lb. Grounded Pork

- 1 tsp. Sea Salt

- 1 cup Parmesan Cheese, shredded

- 2 Eggs

Method of Preparation:

1. Start by cooking the grounded pork until they are browned in a large skillet over medium-high heat.

2. Now, transfer the cooked meat to a large bowl and stir in eggs, cheese, and salt.

3. Give a good mix, and then select the broiler function of the oven.

4. Preheat the broiler to high heat and place a greased parchment-paper-lined baking sheet in the second rack from the top.

5. Next, shape balls out of the meat mixture and arrange them on the baking sheet while leaving ample space in between.

6. Broil them for 4 minutes or until the top portions start getting thickened.

7. Then, change the broiler function to 'bake' mode and bake for 20 to 25 minutes or until cooked.

8. Serve it warm and enjoy.

Tip: If permitted in your diet, you can add dried basil, thyme, and oregano.

Serving Suggestion: The meatballs are delicious on their own. Or you can serve it along with more cheese or cream sauce.

Storage Suggestion: Store the meatballs in an air-tight container in the refrigerator for three to four days.

Nutritional Information per Serving:

- **Calories**: 116Kcal
- **Fat**: 10g
- **Carbohydrates**: 1g
- **Proteins**: 8g

PORK BELLY

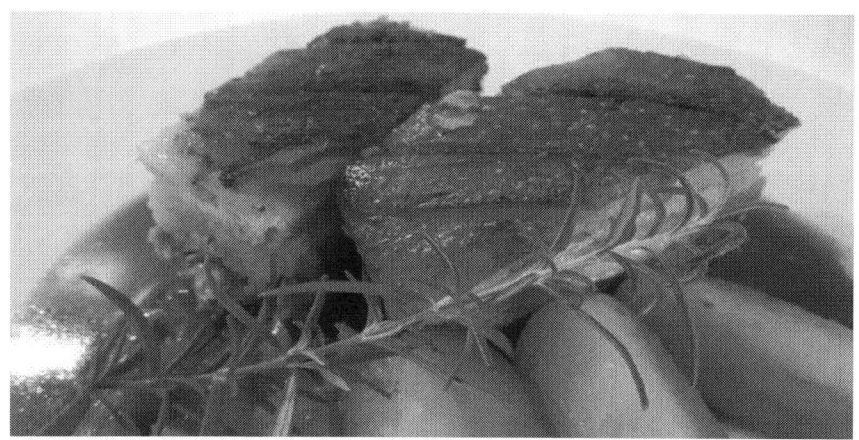

For the perfectly golden brown and crisp crackling pork belly, this easy carnivore-styled recipe is sure to help you. To boot, the incredibly rich pork belly is crispy on the outside while being tender and juicy inside.

Preparation Time: 5 Minutes

Cooking Time: 25 Minutes

Serving Size: 4

Ingredients:

- 2 lb. Pork Belly with skin

- Sea Salt & Black Pepper, as needed

- 2 tbsp. Butter, melted

Method of Preparation:

1. Preheat the oven to 350 ° F or 175 ° C.

2. Make cuts over the skin and the fat portion of the pork belly on the diagonal without cutting the meat. Tip: They should be at least a half an inch difference between the cuts.

3. Now, coat the meat with butter and then season it with salt and pepper. Keep it aside.

4. Next, place the meat on a greased baking sheet with the skin side up.

5. Finally, bake for 2 ½ hours. Once the baking time is up, increase the temperature to 420 ° F or 210 ° C and cook for further 20 minutes. Allow it to cool slightly for 10 to 20 minutes before slicing and serving. Tip: You can cover it with plastic and refrigerate it until chilled for enhancing the flavor.

6. Serve it warm and enjoy.

Tip: If time permits, refrigerate the pork belly overnight once it is seasoned for more flavor.

Serving Suggestion: The pork belly is delicious on its own. Or it can be served with a simple salad for the contrasting texture.

Storage Suggestion: Store the pork belly in an air-tight container in the refrigerator for three to four days.

Nutritional Information per Serving:

- **Calories**: 297Kcal

- **Fat**: 30g

- **Carbohydrates**: 1g

- **Proteins**: 5g

GROUND BEEF CASSEROLE

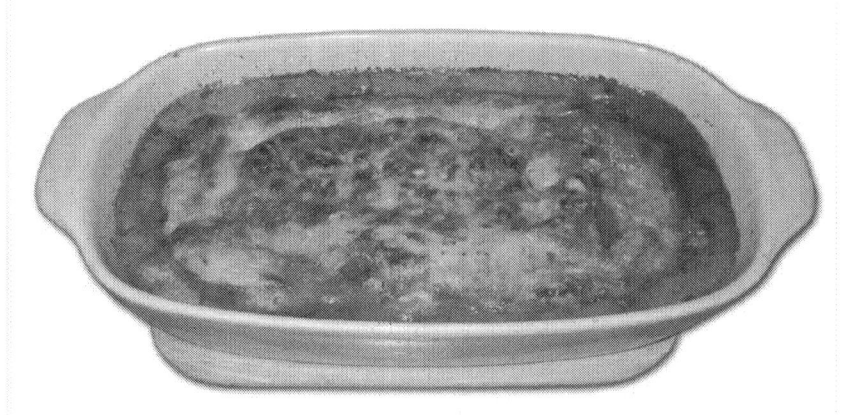

Easy to throw together, this beef casserole is packed with goodness and flavor. Though it is simple to make, it is positively scrumptious, making it a winner wherever it is served.

Preparation Time: 5 Minutes

Cooking Time: 25 Minutes

Serving Size: 4

Ingredients:

- 1 lb. Beef, grounded

- 1 tsp. Sea Salt

- 6 Eggs, large

- 2 tbsp. Cream Cheese, softened

- ½ cup Heavy Cream

- ½ cup Parmesan Cheese, grated

Method of Preparation:

1. Preheat the oven to 350 ° F or 175 ° C.

2. After that, brown the meat in a large skillet over medium-high heat.

3. Next, place the eggs in a large mixing bowl and whisk them well.

4. Then, stir in heavy cream, salt, and cream cheese to it and mix until everything is well incorporated.

5. Now, transfer the mixture to a greased glass plate and top it with the parmesan cheese evenly.

6. Bake for 27 to 30 minutes. Keep it aside for 10 minutes before serving.

7. Serve it warm and enjoy.

Tip: Instead of parmesan cheese, you could also use cheddar cheese or Jack cheese.

Serving Suggestion: The beef casserole is delicious on its own.

Storage Suggestion: Store the beef casserole in an air-tight container in the refrigerator for three to five days.

Nutritional Information per Serving:

- **Calories**: 523Kcal

- **Fat**: 43g

- **Carbohydrates**: 2g

- **Proteins**: 30g

MEAT MUFFINS

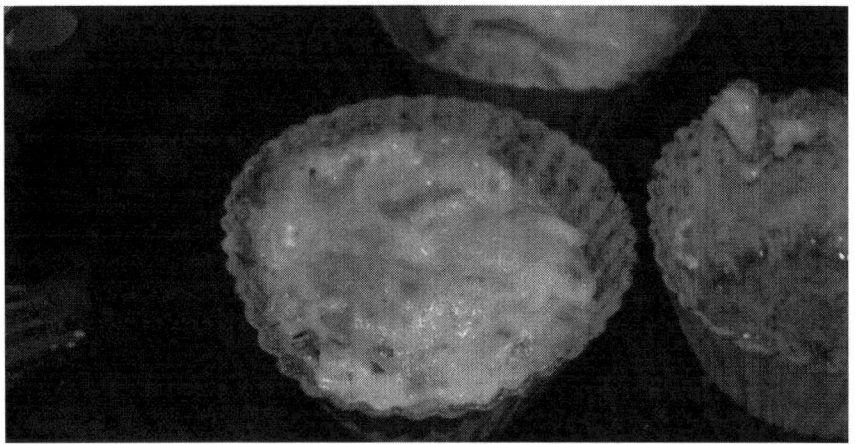

These delicious meat muffins are a great way to enjoy the taste and flavor of the beef liver and eggs. Alongside, the muffins are the most enjoyable meal to cook as organ meat is an excellent source of healing nutrition.

Preparation Time: 10 Minutes

Cooking Time: 20 Minutes

Serving Size: 12

Ingredients:

- ¼ lb. Beef Liver, grounded

- 1 lb. Beef, grounded

- 1 tsp. Salt

- 4 Eggs

- 1 tbsp. Beef Tallow

Method of Preparation:

1. Preheat the oven to 350 ° F or 175 ° C.

2. After that, combine the ground beef and ground liver in a large mixing bowl.

3. Then, pour the eggs over the mixture and mix well.

4. To this, spoon in the salt and give a good stir.

5. Now, spoon in the mixture evenly among the molds of the greased muffin pan.

6. Finally, bake them for 18 to 20 minutes or until cooled. Keep them aside for 10 minutes before serving.

7. Serve it warm and enjoy.

Tip: If you desire, you can soak the liver in ice-cold water to remove the intense taste of the liver.

Serving Suggestion: The meat muffin is delicious on its own. Or you can pair it with sugar-free mayonnaise dip.

Storage Suggestion: Store the meat muffin in an air-tight container in the refrigerator for three to five days.

Nutritional Information per Serving:

- **Calories**: 139Kcal

- **Fat**: 10g

- **Carbohydrates**: 1g

- **Proteins**: 10g

LIVER PATE

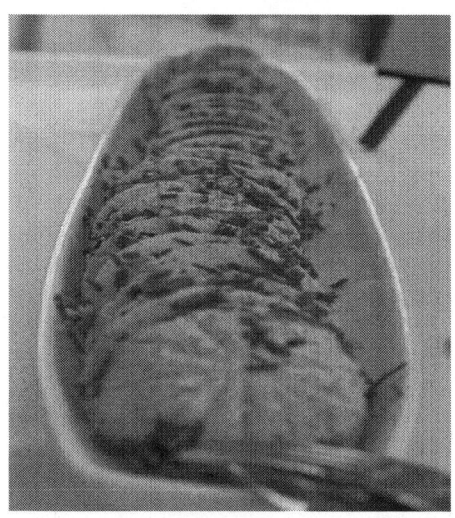

Inexpensive and easy to make, this liver pate dish has a wonderfully smooth texture while having a mild, rich flavor. What's more, the dish has an abundance of flavor which makes it more interesting.

Preparation Time: 10 Minutes

Cooking Time: 10 Minutes

Serving Size: 6

Ingredients:

- ¼ tsp. Black Pepper, grounded

- ½ lb. Chicken Liver

- ½ tsp. Salt

- ½ cup Butter, softened

- ½ tsp. Garlic Powder

- 1 tbsp. Parsley, optional

Method of Preparation:

1. Begin by melting the butter in a large-sized saucepan over medium-high heat, and once it is melted, add the chicken liver pieces.

2. Cook for 7 minutes or until softened.

3. Now, season it with salt, garlic powder, and pepper.

4. Next, transfer the meat mixture to the high-speed to a food processor and grind them for 4 to 5 minutes or until smooth without lumps.

5. Serve and enjoy.

Tip: Liver pate tastes best when served cold.

Serving Suggestion: The liver pate is delicious when served on top of low-carb treats.

Storage Suggestion: Store the liver pate in an air-tight container covered with plastic wring and press in the refrigerator for five days. Topping it with lard makes it last much longer.

Nutritional Information per Serving:

- **Calories**: 139Kcal

- **Fat**: 10g

- **Carbohydrates**: 1g

- **Proteins**: 10g

LAMB CHOPS

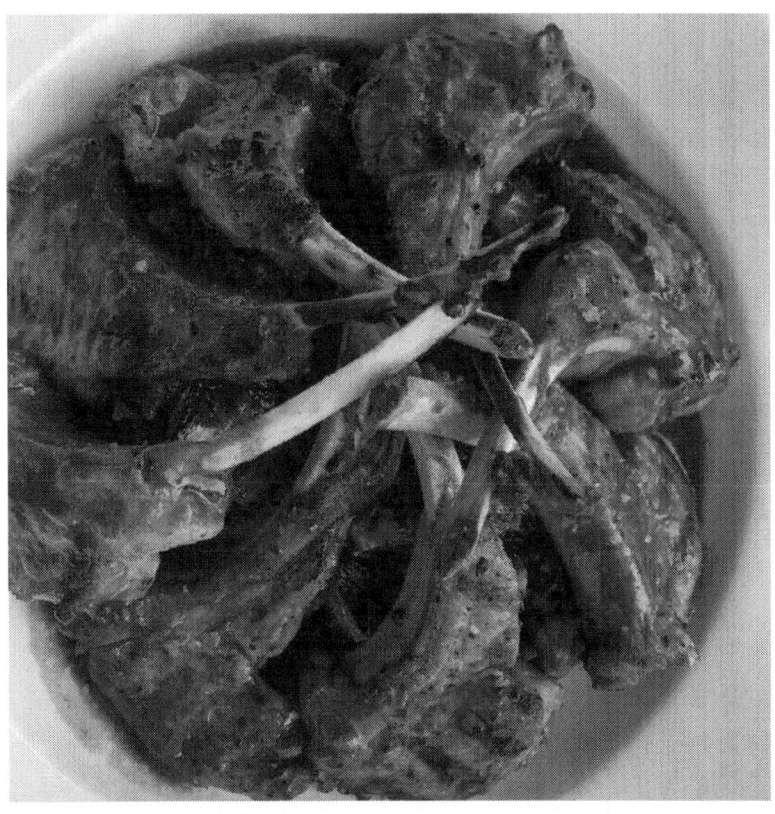

These lamb chops have the simplest yet incredible flavor combo. Between the black pepper, garlic powder, butter, sea salt, your taste buds are sure to tingle. The dish will be one of the most enjoyable food you can make as it has such a tenderizing texture and a uniquely rich, savory flavor, which all will love.

Preparation Time: 10 Minutes

Cooking Time: 10 Minutes

Serving Size: 4

Ingredients:

- 1 tsp. Black Pepper, grounded
- 4 Lamb Shoulder Chops, medium-sized
- ½ tsp. Garlic Powder
- 2 tbsp. Butter
- 1 tsp. Sea Salt
- 1 tsp. Rosemary, dried

Method of Preparation:

1. To start with, combine rosemary, salt, garlic, and pepper in a small bowl and then coat the lamb chops with it.

2. Now, coat it over the lamb chops and allow it to marinate for a minimum of four hours Or overnight.

3. Next, heat a large saucepan over medium heat, and once it is hot, melt the butter and place the chops in it.

4. Cook them for 4 minutes or until it is browned and cooked.

5. Serve it warm and enjoy.

Tip: Based on the strictness of your diet, you can add or spoon in lemon juice to brighten the flavor.

Serving Suggestion: The lamb chops are delicious on their own. Or you can pair it with your favorite salad.

Storage Suggestion: Store the lamb chops in an air-tight container in the refrigerator for three to five days.

Nutritional Information per Serving:

- **Calories**: 358Kcal

- **Fat**: 17.9g

- **Carbohydrates**: 1g

- **Proteins**: 46. 3g

BONE MARROW BROTH

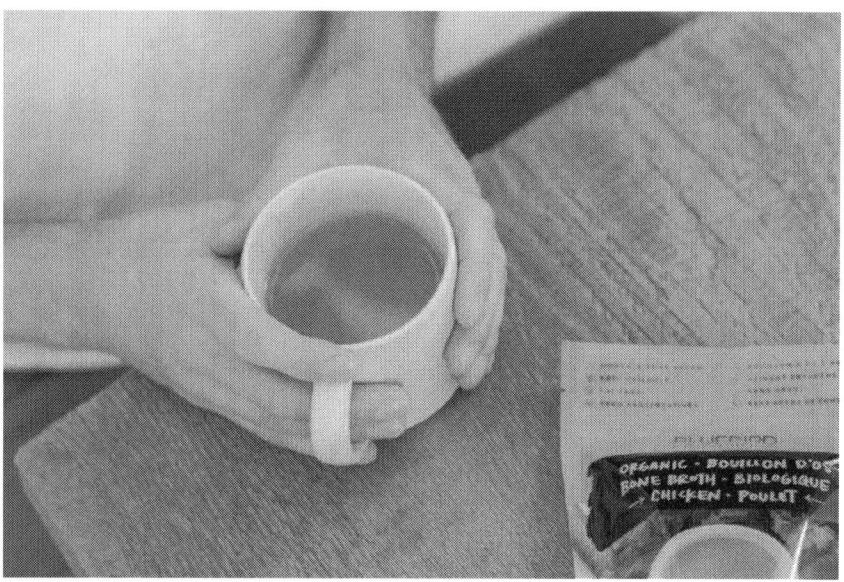

A recipe showing how to make super-flavorful yet simple and nutrient-dense bone marrow is essential to know, especially when following the carnivore diet. On top of it, the broth is so nourishing and refreshing.

Preparation Time: 30 Minutes

Cooking Time: 10 Minutes + 18 Hours

Serving Size: 8

Ingredients:

- ¼ cup Apple Cider Vinegar

- 6 lb. Beef Bones

Method of Preparation:

1. To make this nutrient-dense broth, arrange all the bone

pieces in a large baking pan and bake for 17 to 20 minutes at 450 ° F or 225 ° C.

2. Next, keep the roasted bones in a large pot and pour water into it until the bones are fully covered.

3. Add vinegar and stir well. Bring the mixture to a simmer and later reduce the heat.

4. Cook for 18 hours and ensure that the bones are always covered with water. Tip:

5. Allow it to cool completely before storing.

6. Stain with a filter.

7. Serve it warm and enjoy.

Tip: To remove the fat, you can add ice to the broth to have a healthy broth minus the fat.

Serving Suggestion: The broth can be used in many dishes.

Storage Suggestion: Store the bone marrow broth pate in an air-tight container in the refrigerator for five days. Or you can freeze them in freezer-friendly containers.

Nutritional Information per Serving:

- Calories: 3Kcal

- Fat: 3g

- Carbohydrates: 1g

- Proteins: 1g

EGG SMOKED SALMON CREPES

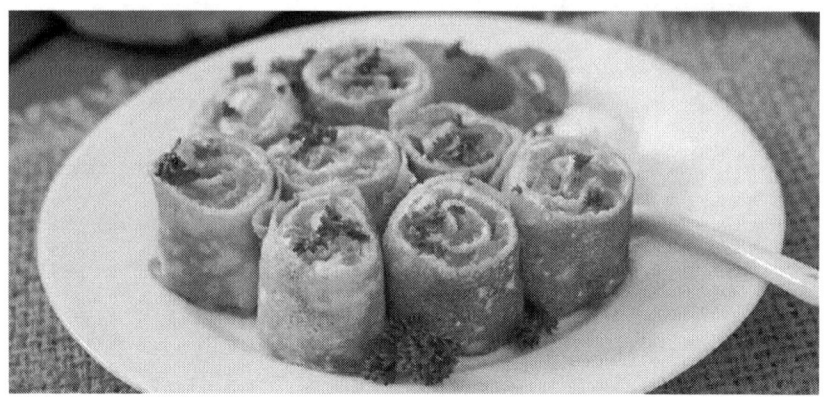

One of the decadent yet healthy ways to kick start your morning is by making these protein-loaded crepes. Furthermore, they are simple to make, healthy, and highly-satiating.

Preparation Time: 10 Minutes

Cooking Time: 10 Minutes

Serving Size: 8

Ingredients:

- Dash of Salt

- 8 Eggs

- 7 oz. Cream Cheese

- Pinch of Dill, optional

- 10 oz. Smoked Salmon

Method of Preparation:

1. Begin by whisking eggs and salt in a large mixing bowl until combined well.

2. After that, heat a medium-sized skillet over medium-high heat, and once it is hot, pour the egg mixture. Swirl it well so that it covers all sides.

3. Cook for a minute or two or until it is set. Flip and cook the other side.

4. Repeat the procedure with the remaining batter.

5. Now, place one crepe on the plate and spread it with cream cheese. Then, spoon in the smoked salmon. Roll the crepe well.

6. Once done, slice it into pieces.

7. Garnish with dill and serve. Enjoy.

Tip: If time permits, place it in the refrigerator for an hour or so.

Serving Suggestion: The egg-smoked salmon crepe is delicious on its own.

Storage Suggestion: Store them in an air-tight container while stacking parchment paper between each of them in the refrigerator for four days.

Nutritional Information per Serving:

- **Calories**: 189Kcal

- **Fat**: 14.2g

- **Carbohydrates**: 1.4g

- **Proteins**: 10.8g

BAKED SALMON

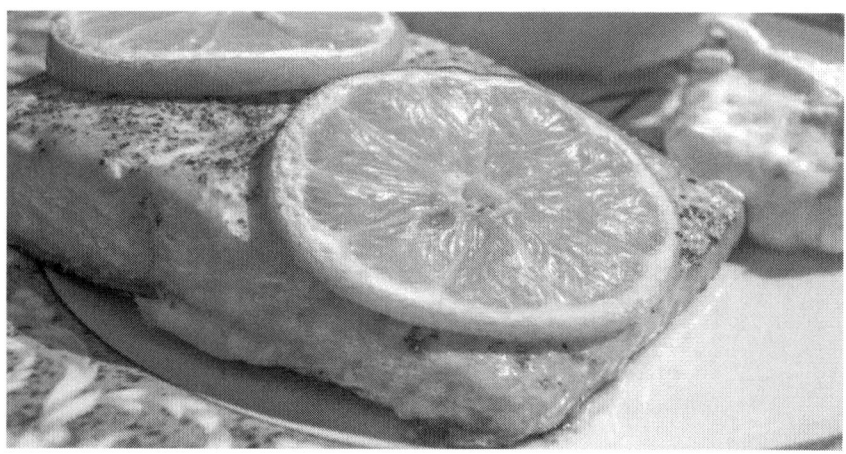

This baked salmon dish contains everything you love about simple fares since it has only minimal ingredients in it. What's more, these simple ingredients make this dish just incredible in its flavor, taste, and texture. Moreover, the baked salmon is juicy and tender insides while having crisp, charred edges.

Preparation Time: 10 Minutes

Cooking Time: 10 Minutes

Serving Size: 4

Ingredients:

- Juice from 1 Lemon

- 1 Salmon Fillet

- Sea Salt, to taste

- Black Pepper, freshly ground, as needed

- 4 Garlic cloves, minced

- 1 tbsp. Butter

Method of Preparation:

1. Preheat the oven to 400 ° F or 200 ° C.

2. Next, keep the salmon on a foil-lined baking sheet with the skin side up.

3. Spoon the lemon juice over the salmon and sprinkle the garlic, salt, and pepper over it.

4. Place butter also on top and bake for 7 to 8 minutes or until cooked.

5. After that, turn on the oven's broiler function and broil the salmon for another 6 to 8 minutes or until it becomes crispy.

6. Serve immediately and enjoy.

Tip: If cilantro is allowed in your diet, you can add about a quarter cup of it to the fare for more flavor.

Serving Suggestion: The baked salmon is delicious on its own. Or you can pair it with lemon butter sauce.

Storage Suggestion: Store them in an air-tight container in the refrigerator for three days.

Nutritional Information per Serving:

- **Calories**: 146Kcal

- **Fat**: 6.9g

- **Carbohydrates**: 2g

- **Proteins**: 19.3g

THREE CHEESE OMELETTE

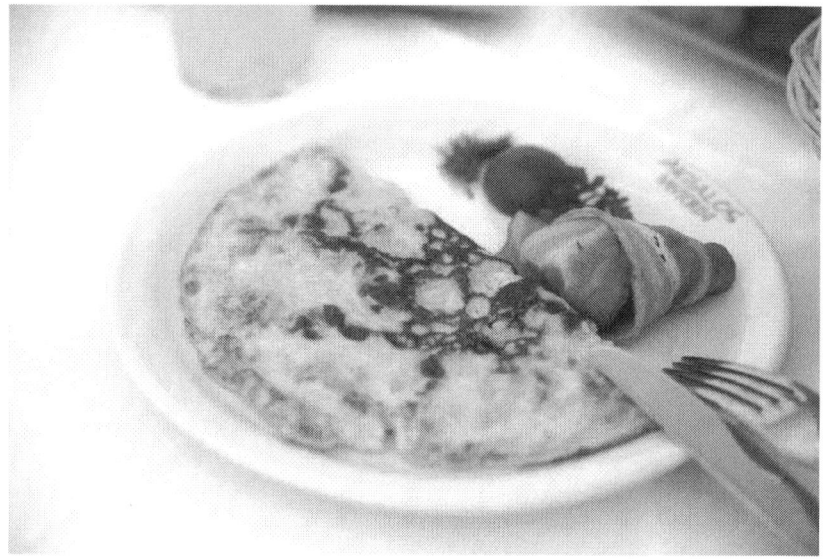

Though this three-cheese omelet looks deceptively simple, it is bursting with flavor and texture. The combo of parmesan cheese, gruyere cheese, and gouda cheese create a hearty, delicious omelet that is also fluffiest and light.

Preparation Time: 10 Minutes

Cooking Time: 5 Minutes

Serving Size: 1

Ingredients:

- 3 Eggs, whole & lightly beaten

- ¼ tsp. Black Pepper, freshly grounded

- ½ tbsp. Butter, preferably grass-fed

- ½ oz. Cheddar Cheese, shredded

- ¼ tsp. Salt

- ½ oz. Gruyere Cheese, shredded

- 1 tbsp. Butter softened

- ½ oz. Gouda Cheese, shredded

Method of Preparation:

1. Heat a large pan over medium-high heat. Once hot, spoon in the butter. Melt the butter.

2. Whisk the eggs along with salt and pepper in a large mixing bowl.

3. Once the butter has melted, transfer the egg mixture to the skillet and keep the shredded cheeses over it in the center portion.

4. Now, allow the eggs to cook and the cheese to become melty and gooey. Fold over.

5. Serve immediately and enjoy.

Tip: If cilantro is allowed in your diet, you can add about a quarter cup of it to the fare for more flavor.

Serving Suggestion: The three-cheese omelet is delicious on its own.

Storage Suggestion: Store them in an air-tight container in the refrigerator for three to five days.

Nutritional Information per Serving:

- **Calories**: 146Kcal

- **Fat**: 6.9g

- **Carbohydrates**: 1g

- **Proteins**: 12g

BUTTER ROASTED CHICKEN

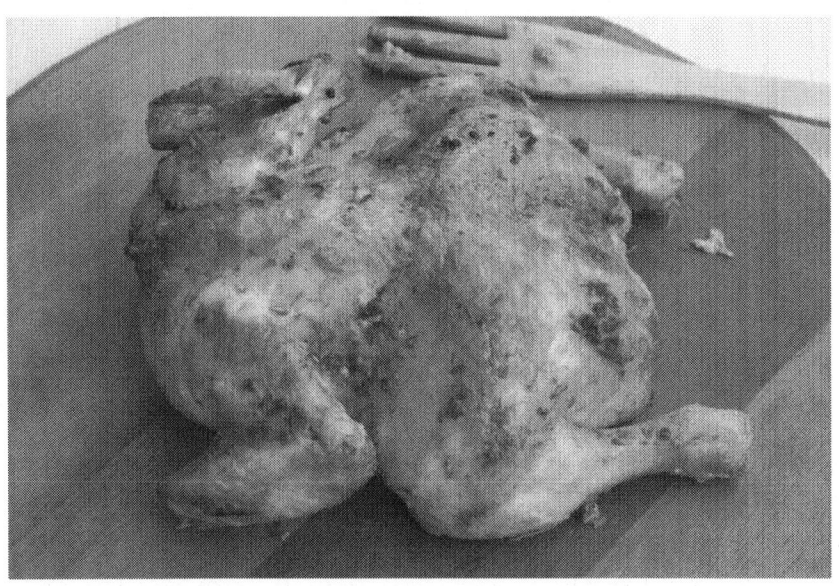

This butter roasted chicken with its crispy chicken and juicy meat is miles apart from the usual roast fare with its unbeatable flavor. What makes it unique is its taste since the butter melts into the chicken and permeates it inside out with a buttery rich flavor.

Preparation Time: 35 Minutes

Cooking Time: 10 Minutes

Serving Size: 6

Ingredients:

- 6 lb. Chicken, whole

- 1 tsp. Garlic, finely chopped

- 1 Lemon , sliced into halves

- Sea Salt & Black Pepper, as needed
- 1 tbsp. Lemon Zest

Method of Preparation:

1. Preheat the oven to 425 ° F or 210 ° C. Remove the giblets from the chicken.

2. Next, season the cavity with the salt and pepper generously and keep the garlic and one lemon halve inside it. Coat well.

3. Then, tie the chicken legs with twine. Now, keep the chicken on a cast-iron skillet.

4. After that, combine butter, lemon zest, and garlic in a small bowl. Pull the skin gently from the chicken and apply the butter mixture all over it while not breaking the skin.

5. Once done, apply the mixture on top of the chicken skin and season with salt and pepper.

6. Finally, cook the chicken for 50 to 55 minutes or until a thermometer inserted in the center reaches 160 ° F.

7. Serve warm and enjoy.

Tip: If the chicken is getting too browned before the baking time is over, cover it with aluminum foil.

Serving Suggestion: The butter roasted chicken is delicious on its own.

Storage Suggestion: Store the chicken in an air-tight container in the refrigerator for two days.

Nutritional Information per Serving:

- **Calories**: 282Kcal
- **Fat**: 21g
- **Carbohydrates**: 1g
- **Proteins**: 19g

CINNAMON BUTTER CHICKEN THIGH

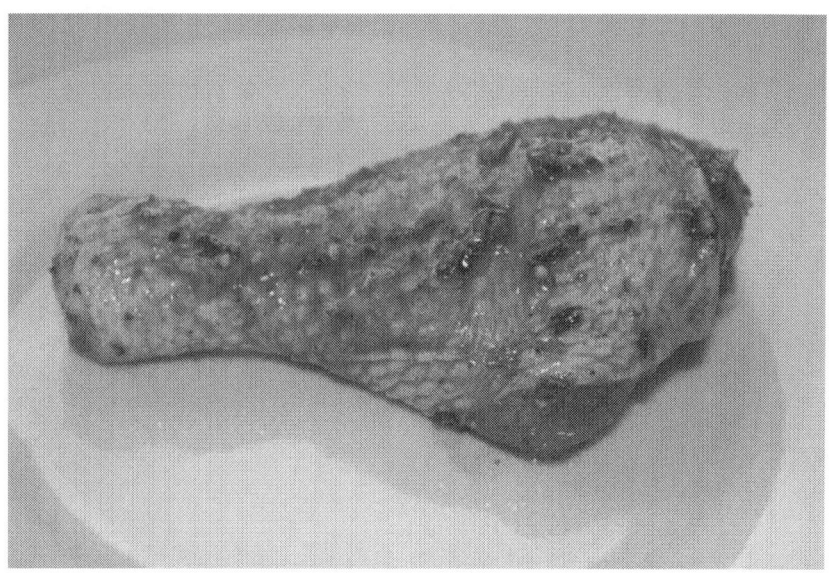

Chicken smothered in cinnamon tanged butter gives this fare its exceptional taste and mind-blowing flavor. Try it, and you are sure to get hooked to it.

Preparation Time: 10 Minutes

Cooking Time: 10 Minutes

Serving Size: 4

Ingredients:

- 2 tsp. Cinnamon, grounded

- 4 Chicken Thighs

- ¼ cup Butter, softened

Method of Preparation:

1. Preheat the oven to 425 ° F or 210 ° C.

2. Next, spoon in the butter to the heated cast-iron skillet over medium heat and once melted, stir in the cinnamon. Mix well. Remove from heat.

3. Now, coat the mixture all over the chicken thighs generously.

4. Return the skillet to the heat and sear the chicken thighs for 4 to 5 minutes or until it is crispy.

5. After that, turn over the chicken and place the skillet in the oven and bake for 20 minutes or until a kitchen thermometer inserted in the center shows 165 ° F.

6. Serve warm and enjoy.

Tip: If the chicken is getting too browned before the baking time is over, cover it with aluminum foil.

Serving Suggestion: The cinnamon butter chicken thigh is delicious on its own.

Storage Suggestion: Store them in an air-tight container in the refrigerator for three to five days.

Nutritional Information per Serving:

- **Calories**: 401Kcal

- **Fat**: 25g

- **Carbohydrates**: 1g

- **Proteins**: 41g

ORGAN MEAT BURGERS

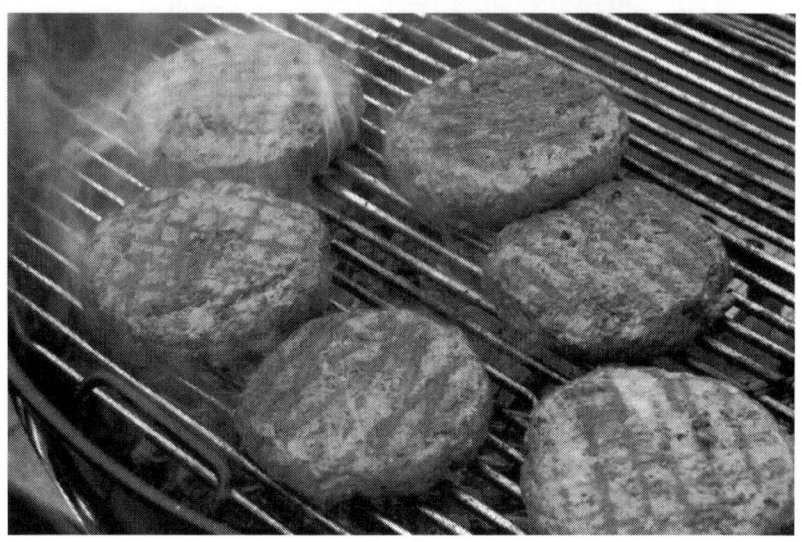

Are you on the lookout for ways to sneak in organ meat for your family? Then, these simple patties should be the first recipe for you to try on since they are so flavorful. Loaded with nutrients, these are highly-satiating while being juicy and tasty.

Preparation Time: 10 Minutes

Cooking Time: 35 Minutes

Serving Size: Makes 15

Ingredients:

- 16 oz. Beef, grounded

- Sea Salt, as required

- 2 Bacon Slices

- 4 oz. Beef Spleen

- 1 tsp. Rosemary, optional

- 4 oz. Beef Kidney

- 1 tbsp. Parsley, optional

Method of Preparation:

- First, place grounded beef, beef kidney, bacon, and beef spleen in a food processor and process for 2 to 3minutes or until you get a meat dough.

- Next, spoon in salt and the seasoning if adding to the dough.

- After that, shape the meat mixture to round patties.

- Then, heat a large saucepan over medium heat and sear each side for about 2 to 2 1/2 minutes or until cooked.

- Serve warm and enjoy.

Tip: If you are planning to freeze, cook the meat 'medium-rare since otherwise, there is a chance for them to overcooked when reheating them.

Serving Suggestion: The organ meat burgers are delicious on their own.

Storage Suggestion: Store them in an air-tight container in the refrigerator for three days.

Nutritional Information per Serving:

- **Calories**: 263Kcal

- **Fat**: 18.1g

- **Carbohydrates**: 3.5g

- **Proteins**: 20.7g

FISH CAKES

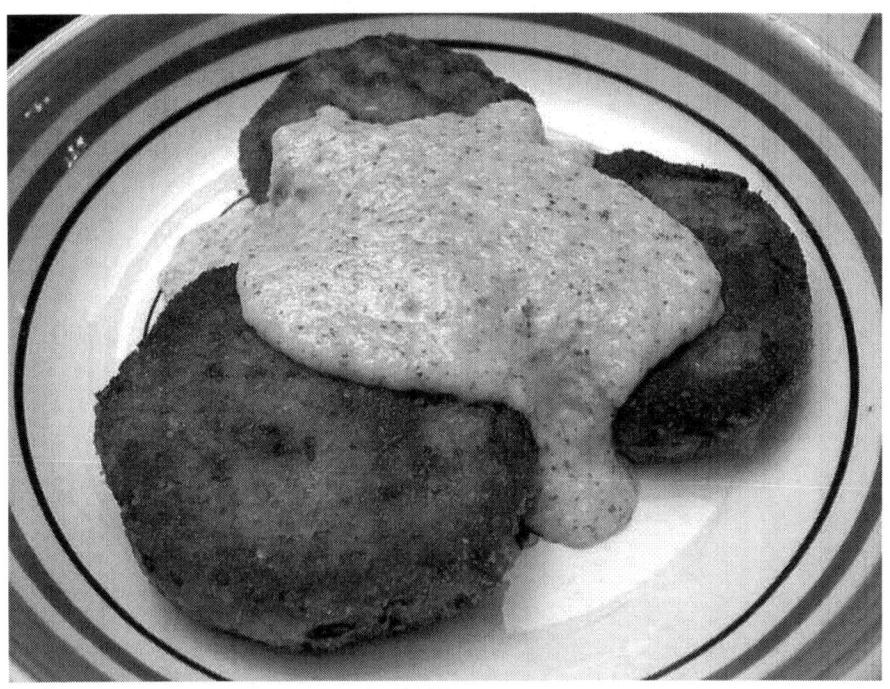

Tasty, crunchy, and delicious, these golden-colored fish cakes are a delight to have with your loved ones. The juicy chunks of the fish inside make these cakes moist and flavorful, making them a winner wherever they are served.

Preparation Time: 10 Minutes

Cooking Time: 60 Minutes

Serving Size: 2

Ingredients:

- ½ lb. Salmon Fillet, skinless & boneless
- 1 Egg
- ½ lb. Smoked Haddock

- 2 tbsp. Butter

- Sea Salt, as needed

- 1 tbsp. Onion Powder

- Black Pepper, as needed

- Cooking Oil, as needed, for frying

Method of Preparation:

1. To start with, chop the salmon and haddock and place them in a large mixing bowl.

2. Next, spoon in the salt, pepper, and garlic powder to it and toss well. O

3. In another bowl, crack the egg and whisk well with a whisker.

4. After that, shape the fish mixture into patties and keep them in the refrigerator for an hour or until chilled.

5. Then, heat a large frying pan and pour oil into it.

6. Finally, fry them for 3 to 4 minutes per side or until just cooked and is golden in color.

7. You can also bake them for 10 minutes in the oven at 320 ° F or 160 ° C for a crunchier coating.

8. Serve warm and enjoy.

Tip: If desired, you can add thyme and parsley for more flavor.

Serving Suggestion: The fish cakes are delicious on their own. Or they can pair along with mayonnaise or goat cheese.

Storage Suggestion: Store them in an air-tight container in the refrigerator for five to seven days.

Nutritional Information per Serving:

- **Calories**: 173Kcal
- **Fat**: 9g
- **Carbohydrates**: 3.5g
- **Proteins**: 15g

BAKED FISH

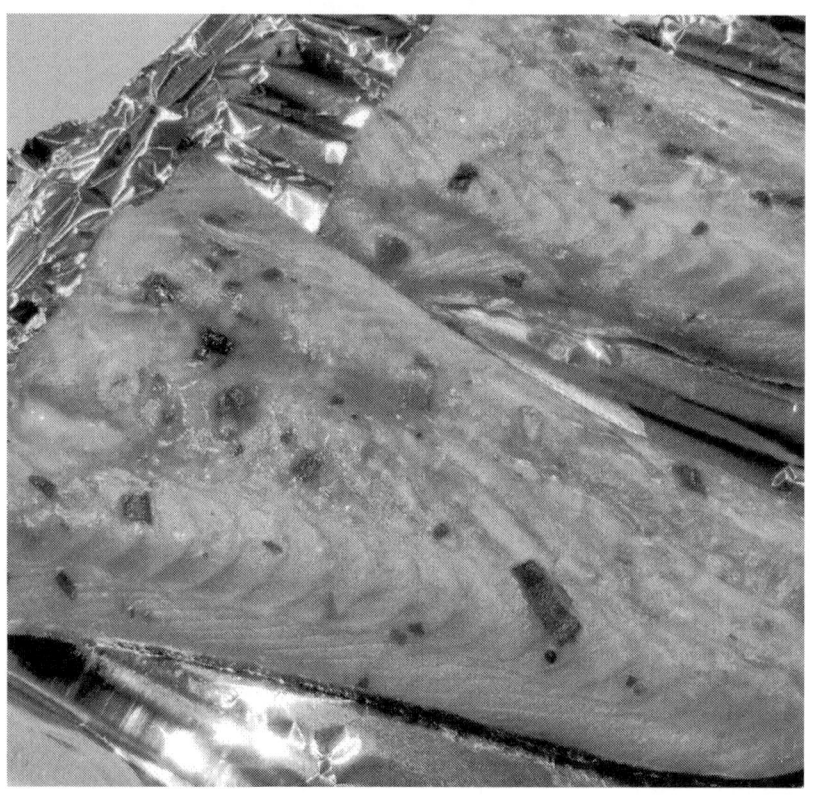

Tender, juicy baked fish in a creamy sauce is a show-stopper wherever you serve them. Furthermore, the combo of fish with parmesan cheese and heavy cream makes it a match made in heaven.

Preparation Time: 10 Minutes

Cooking Time: 60 Minutes

Serving Size: 4

Ingredients:

- 2 tbsp. Garlic Powder, optional
- 1 cup Parmesan Cheese, shredded
- 1 ½ lb. White Fish Fillets, washed, dried & patted
- Sea Salt, as needed
- 1 ½ cup Heavy Cream

Method of Preparation:

1. First, heat the oven to 350 ° F or 175 ° C.
2. Next, season the fish fillets with salt and onion powder. Set it aside.
3. Then, combine half of the heavy cream and parmesan cheese in another bowl with a whisker and whisk well.
4. Now, dip the fish fillets in the mixture and coat well on all sides.
5. After that, bake the fillets for 20 minutes or until cooked.
6. Once twenty minutes have passed, coat them with the remaining parmesan and bake for further 1o minutes.
7. Serve warm and enjoy.

Tip: You can either use evaporated milk instead of heavy cream.

Serving Suggestion: The baked fish is delicious on its own. Or they can pair along with the lemon cream sauce.

Storage Suggestion: Store them in an air-tight container in the refrigerator for two to three days.

Nutritional Information per Serving:

- **Calories**: 341Kcal
- **Fat**: 16g
- **Carbohydrates**: 1g
- **Proteins**: 33g

GRILLED TUNA

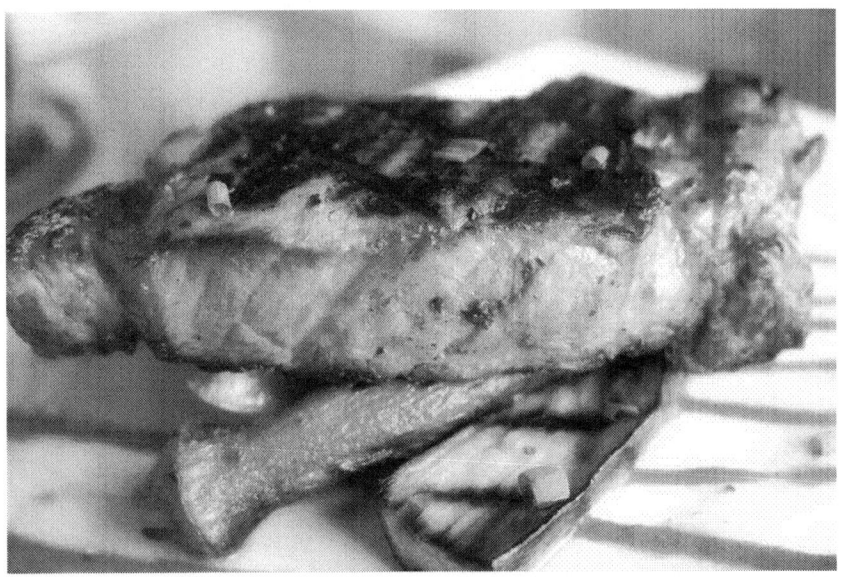

Enjoying the flavor of tuna fish becomes so much easier with this simple yet quick recipe. Perfectly seared on the outside while having juicy insides makes this grilled seafood is a good change from the grilled meats.

Preparation Time: 10 Minutes

Cooking Time: 35 Minutes

Serving Size: 4

Ingredients:

- 4 Tuna

- Sea Salt & Black Pepper, as required

- 2 tbsp. Lemon Juice

Method of Preparation:

1. For making this easy seafood fare, heat the grill to high.

2. After that, season the tuna with salt and pepper. Set aside for a few minutes.

3. Next, place them on the heated grill and cook them for 2 to 3 minutes or until they are cooked to your desired done level.

4. Allow the fish to cool for 10 to 15 minutes before slicing.

5. Serve warm and enjoy.

Tip: Frozen tuna works well for this recipe.

Serving Suggestion: The grilled tuna are delicious on their own.

Storage Suggestion: Store them in an air-tight container in the refrigerator for two days.

Nutritional Information per Serving:

- **Calories**: 93Kcal

- **Fat**: 2g

- **Carbohydrates**: 0g

- **Proteins**: 20.8g

STIR-FRIED BEEF HEARTS

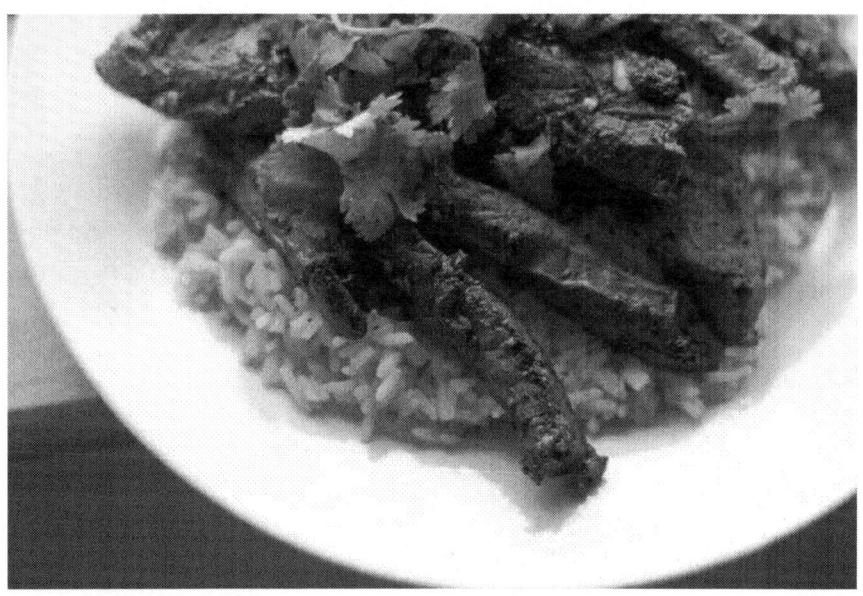

Once you are getting accustomed to the carnivore diet, this recipe for stir-fried beef hearts should be the first one to try out. In fact, you will get surprised by its delightful taste and texture.

Preparation Time: 10 Minutes

Cooking Time: 35 Minutes

Serving Size: 4

Ingredients:

- 2 lb.Beef Hearts

- Sea Salt & Black Pepper, as needed

- 4 tbsp. Butter

- ½ cup Balsamic Vinegar

Method of Preparation:

1. First, wash the fish well and pat it dry. Now, brush it with the vinegar and allow it to marinate overnight.

2. Then, heat a large skillet over medium-high heat, and to this, spoon in the butter.

3. Once the butter has melted, stir in the liver hearts. Season it with salt and pepper. Cook for 3 to 4 minutes or until the meat is browned.

4. Allow it to cool and serve.

Tip: If you prefer a more robust flavor, you can cook for 4 to 5 minutes.

Serving Suggestion: The stir-fried beef hearts are delicious on their own. Or you can pair it with cauliflower rice.

Storage Suggestion: Store them in an air-tight container in the refrigerator for three to four days.

Nutritional Information per Serving:

- **Calories**: 93 Kcal

- **Fat**: 2g

- **Carbohydrates**: 0g

- **Protein**

FOODS ALLOWED ON THE CARNIVORE DIET

Consuming animal products makes your weekly grocery shopping extremely easy. One of the significant advantages of the carnivore diet is how easy it is to follow.

The permitted items on the carnivore diet are:

- **Meat**: All your calorie requirements should come from fatty cuts of grass-fed meat like NY strip steak, porterhouse, ribeye, 80/20 ground beef, t-bone, bacon, pork chops, and flank steak. Since you're curbing carbohydrates, meats with more fat content are preferred so your body can use those fats as a source of energy.

- **Fish**: Look for the fattiest fish you can have, like salmon, sardines, trout, mackerel, and catfish.

- **Eggs:** Called nature's multivitamin, eggs have the ideal ratio of protein, fats, and essential nutrients to keep your body at its optimal best.

- **Bone marrow**: Bone broth is an excellent protein source that aids with gut, skin, and joint health.

- **Dairy**: Milk, grass-fed butter, and cheese as we get them from animals. Dairy is the one grey area within the carnivore diet. Most carnivore dieters exclude dairy products entirely, as many people have unidentified underlying intolerances often associated with lactose or casein. On the 0ther hand, there are carnivore dieters advocates who believe that it should be included because dairy comes from animal-based sources.

- **Lard and other animal-based fats**: Consume lard,

tallow, and other animal-based fats to avoid vegetable oils.

- **Simple spices, seasonings, and condiments**: Salt, pepper, herbs, and spices are permissible on the carnivore diet. Select simple ingredients that don't encompass any sugar or carbohydrates. If you prefer the flavor, consider adding some zero-calorie hot sauce like Frank's Red Hot.

- Processed Meats: You can eat processed cold meats like ham, salami, chorizo, & pepperoni. However, they are best dodged for the first month if possible. This is because you may be eating extra carbohydrate fillers mistakenly with these types of deli meats.

FOODS TO AVOID ON THE CARNIVORE DIET

Adopting the carnivore diet is highly restrictive, so that means most of your usual snacks and meals would be eliminated. Though it will be a bit overwhelming, you will start feeling better with time.

Here's what you can't have on carnivore:

- Fruits: Apples, bananas, berries, mangoes, etc.

- Vegetables: All vegetables also involve vegetable stock and any condiments made from vegetables.

- Sugars: Added sugars across the board are not permitted! It is true also for natural-based sugars as well.

- All Preservatives: Processed foods include nitrates, nitrites, MSG, and other additives typically seen in frozen and canned food.

- Poor-Quality meat: Even though the carnivore diet is meat-based, that doesn't mean any beef is on the table. To avoid the inflammation caused by grain, you need to eat grass-fed and pasture-raised meats.

- Grains: No bread or grains of any kind are allowed in the carnivore diet. This means o rice, no pasta, all nuts, seeds, and legumes:

- Nuts, grains, and legumes shouldn't be taken. Almonds, peanuts, peas, flax seeds, chia seeds, etc.

3 DAY MEAL PLAN

Day 1:

Breakfast – Poached Egg (Calories 138 Fat 10g; Proteins 1g; Carbs 1.3g)

Lunch: Pork Chops (Calories 399; Fat 10g; Proteins 46g; Carbs 2g)

Dinner: Ground Beef Casserole (Calories 523, Fat 43g; Proteins 30g; Carbs 2g)

Total: 1060 Calories; Fat 63g; Proteins 77g; Carbohydrates 5.3g

Day 2:

Breakfast: Scotch Egg (Calories 458; Fat 30g; Proteins 45g; Carbs 2g)

Lunch: Lamb Chops (Calories 358; Fat 17.9g; Proteins 46.1g; Carbs 3g)

Dinner: Pickled Egg (Calories 85.5; Fat 10g; Proteins 8g; Carbs 1g)

Total: 901.5Calories, Fat 57.9g; Proteins 99.1g; Carbohydrates 6g

Day 3:

Breakfast: Egg Omelette (Calories 458; Fat 30g; Proteins 45g; Carbs 1g)

Lunch: Baked Salmon (Calories 146; Fat 6.9g; Proteins 19.3g; Carbs 2g)

Dinner: Deli Roast Beef (Calories 452; Fat 30g; Proteins 43g; Carbs 2g)

Total: 665Calories, Fat 66.9g; Proteins 107.3g; Carbs 5g)

7 DAY MEAL PLAN

Day 1:

Breakfast – Carnivore Waffles (Calories 270; Fat 19g; Proteins 24.7g; Carbs 1.3g)

Lunch: Pork Chops (Calories 399; Fat 10g; Proteins 46g; Carbs 2g)

Dinner: Ground Beef Casserole (Calories 523, Fat 43g; Proteins 30g; Carbs 2g)

Total: 1192 Calories; Fat 72g; Proteins 100.7g; Carbohydrates 5.3g

Day 2:

Breakfast: Egg Omelette (Calories 458; Fat 30g; Proteins 45g; Carbs 2g)

Lunch: Lamb Chops (Calories 358; Fat 17.9g; Proteins 46.1g; Carbs 3g

Dinner: Meatballs (Calories 116; Fat 10g; Proteins 8g; Carbs 1g)

Total: 932Calories, Fat 57.9g; Proteins 99.1g; Carbohydrates 6g

Day 3:

Breakfast: Three Cheese Omelette (Calories 222; Fat 19g; Proteins 12g; Carbs 1g)

Lunch: Pork Belly (Calories 297; Fat 30g; Proteins 5g; Carbs 1g)

Dinner: Baked Salmon (Calories 146; Fat 6.9g; Proteins 19.3g; Carbs 2g)

Total: 665Calories, Fat 55.9g; Proteins 36.3g; Carbs 4g)

Day 4:

Breakfast – Ham & Goat Cheese Frittata (Calories 290; Fat 22g; Proteins 20g; Carbs 0.5g)

Lunch: Butter Roasted Chicken (Calories 282; Fat 21g; Proteins 19g; Carbs 1g)

Dinner: Chicken Wings (Calories 348, Fat 27g; Proteins 25g; Carbs 1g)

Total: 920 Calories; Fat 70g; Proteins 100.7g; Carbohydrates 2.5g

Day 5:

Breakfast: Baked Ham & Egg (Calories 340; Fat 30g; Proteins 13g; Carbs 3g)

Lunch: Scotch Eggs (Calories 270; Fat 20g; Proteins 19g; Carbs 1g)

Dinner: Carnivore Custard (Calories 420; Fat 44g; Proteins 4g; Carbs 3g)

Total: 1030Calories, Fat 94g; Proteins 36g; Carbohydrates 7g

Day 6:

Breakfast: Bacon Egg Quiche (Calories 310; Fat 26g; Proteins 17g; Carbs 2g)

Lunch: Deli Roast Beef (Calories 452; Fat 30g; Proteins 43g; Carbs 0g)

Dinner: Cinnamon Butter Chicken Thigh (Calories 401; Fat 25g; Proteins 41g; Carbs 1g)

Total: 1163Calories, Fat 81g; Proteins 101g; Carbs 3g

Day 7:

Breakfast: Meat Muffins (Calories 139; Fat 10g; Proteins 10g; Carbs 1g)

Lunch: Butter Burger (Calories 125; Fat 10g; Proteins 8g; Carbs 0g)

Dinner: Egg Smoked Salmon Crepes (Calories 189; Fat 14.2g; Proteins 10.8g; Carbs 1.4g)

Total: 592Calories, Fat 34.2g; Proteins 28.8g; Carbs 2.4g)

THANK YOU
FOR FINISHING THE BOOK!

We would like to thank you very much for supporting us and reading through to the end. We know you could have picked any number of books to read, but you picked this book and for that, we are extremely grateful.

We hope you enjoyed your reading experience. If so, it would be really nice if you could share this book with your friends and family by posting on Facebook and Twitter.

Delicious Delights Publishing stands for the highest reading quality and we will always endeavor to provide you with high-quality books.

Would you mind leaving us a review on Amazon before you go? Because it will mean a lot to us and support us in creating high-quality guidelines for you in the future.

Please help us reach more readers by taking 30 seconds to write just a few words on Amazon now

(https://www.amazon.com/review/create-review/ref=cm_cr_othr_d_wr_but_top?ie=UTF8&channel=glance-detail&asin=B09C13KGFR)

Warmly yours,

The Delicious Delights Publishing Team

IF YOU'VE ENJOYED
THE FRUGAL CARNIVORE DIET MADE EASY,
YOU'LL ALSO ENJOY IN THIS SERIES:

HOME DISTILLATION FOR BEGINNERS:

Find out how to Distill Spirits Easily and What Equipment You
Need For Your Home Distillery

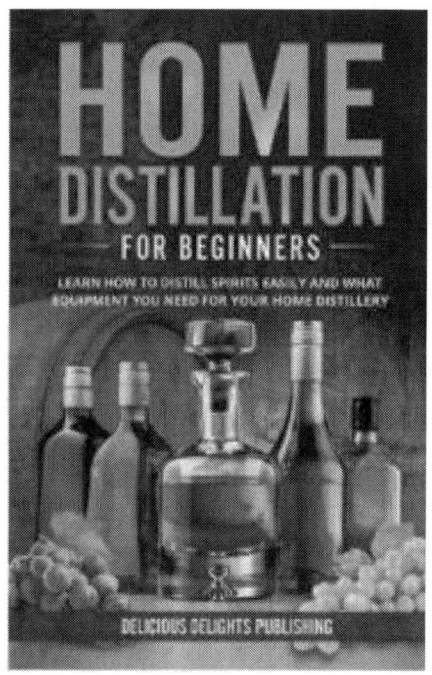

https://amzn.to/3rYNNg6*

GROWING HERBS FOR BEGINNERS:

How to Grow Herbs Indoors in Pots and Outdoors in Planter

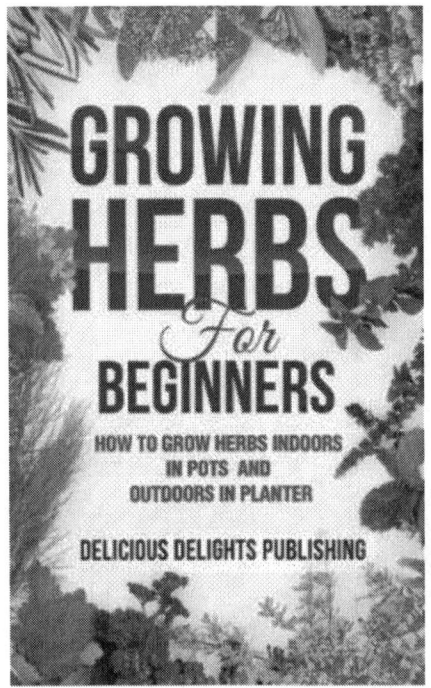

https://amzn.to/3e6LFOf*

VEGAN SAUCES MADE EASY:

35 Tasty and Healthy Popular Vegan Sauce Recipes

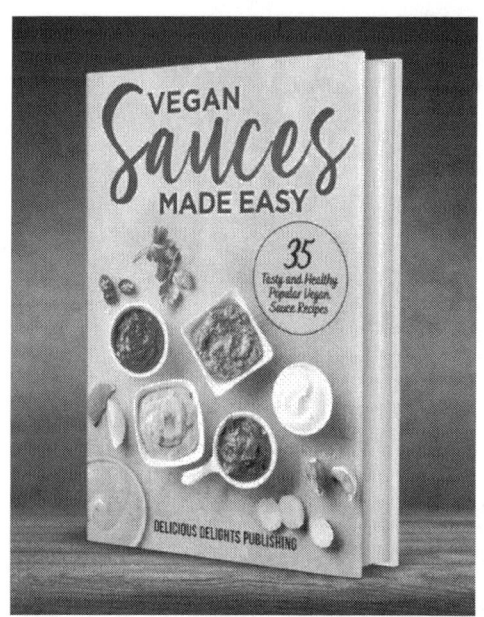

https://www.amazon.com/dp/B095GFBZLH

THE ULTIMATE MACARON BAKING COOKBOOK FOR BEGINNERS:

How to Make Colorful Macarons Easily

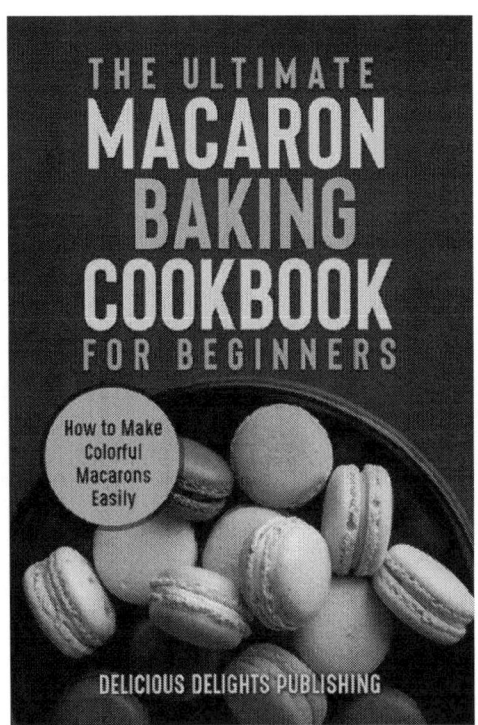

https://www.amazon.com/dp/B097SQQSSY

The links marked with an asterisk (*) are so-called affiliate links. If you click on such an affiliate link and shop via this link, I will receive a commission from the online shop or provider concerned. For you, the price doesn't change.

Thank you!

32936693R00052